Too Old for Health Care?

The Johns Hopkins Series in Contemporary Medicine and Public Health

Also of Interest in This Series:

William Halsey Barker, M.D., *Adding Life to Years: Organized Geriatrics Services in Great Britain and Implications for the United States*

James E. Birren and Donna E. Deutchman, *Guiding Autobiography Groups for Older Adults: Exploring the Fabric of Life*

Carl Eisdorfer, PH.D., M.D., David A. Kessler, M.D., J.D., and Abby N. Spector, M.M.H.S., eds., *Caring for the Elderly: Reshaping Health Policy*

Madelon Lubin Finkel and Hirsch S. Ruchlin, *The Health Care Benefits of Retirees*

Vincent Mor, PH.D., David S. Greer, M.D., and Robert Kastenbaum, PH.D., eds., *The Hospice Experiment*

William G. Weissert, Jennifer M. Elston, Elise J. Bolda, William N. Zelman, Elizabeth Mutran, and Anne B. Mangum, *Adult Day Care: Findings from a National Survey*

Too Old for Health Care?

Controversies in Medicine, Law, Economics, and Ethics

Edited by
ROBERT H. BINSTOCK
and
STEPHEN G. POST

with the assistance of
LAUREL S. MILLS

THE JOHNS HOPKINS UNIVERSITY PRESS
Baltimore and London

The Johns Hopkins University Press
701 West 40th Street
Baltimore, Maryland 21211
The Johns Hopkins Press Ltd., London

The paper used in this book meets
the minimum requirements of American
National Standard for Information
Sciences—Permanence of Paper for Printed
Library Materials, ANSI Z39.48-1984.

Library of Congress Cataloging-in-Publication Data

Too old for health care? : controversies in medicine,
law, economics, and ethics/edited by Robert H.
Binstock and Stephen G. Post; with the assistance of
Laurel S. Mills.
        p.   cm.—(The Johns Hopkins series in
contemporary medicine and public health)
    Includes bibliographical references and index.
    ISBN 0-8018-4165-8 (alk. paper).—
    ISBN 0-8018-4248-4 (pbk.)
    1. Aged—Medical care—United States.
2. Medical ethics—United States. 3. Medical care,
Cost of—United States. I. Binstock, Robert H.
II. Post, Stephen Garrard, 1951–   . III. Mills,
Laurel S. IV. Series.
RA564.8.T66   1991
362.1′9897′00973—dc20   90-23237 CIP

Contents

Foreword

There could have been another surgeon general's warning: "Warning! The American health care system can be hazardous to your health."

Costs are escalating; some hospital emergency rooms and doctors' offices are overcrowded; high-tech medicine is prolonging the lives of terminally ill patients at outrageous expense and often against the family's will; medical staffs are overworked and burnt out; medical school applications are leveling off after a downward spiral, while the costs of medical malpractice insurance are soaring in the opposite direction.

We are clearly in the midst of a health care crisis. This is not to say that the medical advancements we have made over the years are not enviable. They are magnificent. As a measure of this success, we now enjoy an average life expectancy of eighty-two years. But, with every advancement comes a trade-off, and the graying of America is undoubtedly an additional burden on an already strained health economy. This book puts into perspective the ethical, moral, social, and legal issues regarding the health care of elderly people.

The trend is clear. By the year 2005, 35 million Americans will be over sixty-five years of age. The largest segment of that population—50 percent—will be persons over seventy-five, so it is expected that by 2005 we will see 100,000 people celebrating a 100th birthday. The implications for our society are serious, and we need to make prudent decisions about the future. On the one hand, we can't minimize the problem, but, on the other, we can't victimize aging people and say the expedient way is the only way out.

Stereotypes of elderly people are changing as senior citizens compete with young people for a bigger piece of a shrinking pie. Once believed to be poor, frail, defenseless victims of a wasteful nation, some of our senior citizens are now seen as affluent, healthy, active, and able to care for themselves. If they accept assistance from the government, they are viewed as "selfish." In other words, they are hardly needy, and by taking advantage of a nation's generosity, they have become an additional economic burden on society.

We can't let this view blur the larger picture, which includes that portion of the elderly population for whom Social Security and Medicare are, quite literally, life savers. Medicare is one of the most decent things this country has done to remove much of the fear and uncertainty from the frail years of elderly life, and it should stand as a landmark of the basic decency of the American ethical core. But it needs to work as originally intended and promised.

So, what can be done? Federal programs are exhausted and/or inefficient, but costs keep going up and more and more people will be in need of services. More regulation won't work. As it stands now, the administration of health care consumes about 22 percent of health care spending. It is my belief that cost containment cannot be achieved if that alone is the goal; rather, costs will be contained only if we focus on high-efficiency and high-quality medical care and reward those who provide it with more patients and not with more money, as we do now.

The other possible solution that inevitably turns up in a discussion about how to fix our health care system is *rationing*. Yet, while many Americans fear the talk of inevitable rationing, they fail to recognize that rationing is already with us. It came about without any dialogue, because of the gap between our aspirations for health care and our resources to pay for it. And so there are emerging from this state of panic some shrill voices—and some less shrill—expressing a desire for some kind of a consensus about decisions that have to be made at the end of life. We hear the suggestion that, at the most, elderly people have an obligation to die, or, at the very least, their health care should be limited. Personally, I feel that many of these voices are misinterpreted. Reading what an author has actually written, as opposed to what the headline editors or critics write, can often provide a more complete understanding of a set of ideas. Daniel Callahan, for example, is one who is more compassionate and less rigid than his critics paint him. However, I do disagree sharply when he defines rationing based on age alone.

Age is far too loose a criterion. Look at me. One of the main reasons I was rebuffed during my nomination to the office of surgeon general was because I was "too old." I was just a youngster of sixty-five. But all my critics said that sixty-five was the age at which surgeons general were supposed to *leave* the public health service, not enter it for the first time. Of course, this did not sit very well with the man who nominated me. President Reagan had just passed his seventieth birthday and did not take kindly to the idea that someone five years his junior was too old for public service.

So it goes with health care. One sixty-five-year-old may not be the same as another sixty-five-year-old. Should both forego an operation to make room for a forty-five-year-old with potentially more productive years to live?

Medical decisions should be based on all factors, *including* age, but not on age alone. A total knee replacement in itself is a marvelous therapeutic advance. But, the function of that knee will depend upon the ability of the individual to undergo strenuous rehabilitation and develop specific muscles to make that knee work. If the patient is frail enough that this kind of rehabilitation is not possible or expected, then the procedure is a waste of scarce resources and should not be done.

I also think it would be wise if we gave more thought to how we can maintain the independence of elderly people. We don't have a means of providing an hour of health care and an hour of chores—such as shopping, cleaning, etc.—for people who are recipients of Medicare or Medicaid. By keeping them independent at a very small expenditure per day, we could keep them out of a nursing home at an exorbitant fee per month.

Instead, our system rewards—with insurance payments—the high-tech medical remedies that kick into place only when the situation is dire. Even now, physicians and patients are debating the wisdom of high-tech care. Elderly people fear it. Their families view it as a mixed blessing, allowing their loved ones to continue living but calling into question the quality of that life, especially at such great monetary and human cost. No matter what financial constraints, we must not let our economics guide our ethics, but must let our ethics guide our economics. We must also be wary of those who are too willing to end the lives of elderly or ill people. If we ever decide that a poor quality of life justifies ending that life, we have taken a step down a slippery slope that places all of us in danger. Medicine cannot be both our healer and our killer.

I find, though, as I travel about the country, that some Americans have forgotten that they have to die—of something. In our society, we shy away from even talking about death. We need to be more realistic. Part of living is preparing for death. Sometimes the most reasonable thing a physician can do for a patient with a terminal illness is to step back and let nature take its course. That is not enthanasia. There is a difference between allowing nature to take its course and actively assisting death.

As the American population ages, these issues will grow in importance. Hospice care of terminally ill people deserves more attention. We must keep our elderly people living as well as they can until they die, and assure them—and ourselves—of a death as free of pain as possible, among friends, a death with serenity.

The content of each of the essays in this book is food for thought. Although I may not agree with everything in every essay, and might disagree sharply with some points in some essays, it still is the basis of enlightenment for people to come to some considered judgment over the course of the next few years.

I offer one closing admonition: Be careful! Your decisions about someone else's life might affect your own sooner than you think.

C. EVERETT KOOP, M.D., SC.D.
Surgeon General, United States Public Health Service
1981–1989

Preface

The foreboding specter of the rationing of health care for people in old age gained widespread attention in U.S. public discourse during the late 1980s. One biomedical ethicist even went so far as to propose that life-saving health care should be denied to a broad category of American citizens, persons in their late seventies or older.

This book is a rejection of such proposals and a source of positive suggestions for dealing with the challenges of health care for our aging society. It is also a wide-ranging analysis of medical, economic, legal, and humanistic issues evoked by the specter of the rationing of health care.

The authors of this volume, though disparate in their professions, in their scholarly disciplines, and in many of their views, are unified by the principle that it is wrong—morally and ethically—to forbid lifesaving care to older persons or to any group categorically, on the basis of demographic characteristics, rather than case by case, on the basis of the individual's clinical condition.

Controversial implications of the proposals for rationing are explored from the perspectives of medicine, law, economics, bioethics, public policy, religion, and the humanities. Gerontologists and geriatricians, as well as professionals in law, ethics, public policy, philosophy, religious studies, the social sciences, the humanities, and health care (e.g., physicians, nurses, social workers, and administrators), will find this book illuminating, stimulating, and practical.

Laypersons will find the book to be interesting, as well, because public proposals for rationing are laden with misperceptions and unnecessary assumptions. This volume presents some of the realities of how health care is provided for elderly people, and how money is spent on various kinds of care. It offers perspectives for considering whether the high costs of health care must inevitably lead to rationing on the basis of demographic categories.

In creating this book, we had support and assistance from a number of organizations and individuals. As we acknowledge them, we also express our appreciation.

The Retirement Research Foundation, of Park Ridge, Illinois, supported the development of this manuscript through a grant award. The National Institute on Aging, of the National Institutes of Health, provided supplementary financial assistance. Case Western Reserve University contributed some faculty time and indirect expenses.

A. Jean Lesher, then executive editor at Scott, Foresman and Company, envisioned the value of this book early in 1989. During the subsequent year, she guided us through the development and completion of it, with exceptional wisdom.

A number of professional colleagues—Kenneth Brummel-Smith, M.D., of the University of Southern California; Patrick J. Fox, Ph.D., of the University of California at San Francisco; Linda George, Ph.D., of Duke University; Robert L. Kane, M.D., of the University of Minnesota; and Mary Joy Quinn, court investigator in San Francisco—undertook critical reviews of all or parts of a draft of the manuscript. We found that their suggestions for changes were extremely thoughtful and valuable as we undertook revisions. We, and the other contributors, are responsible, of course, for the final content of this volume.

Our fellow contributors were exemplary in the quality of their work, their sense of professional responsibility, and their collegiality.

Laurel S. Mills, a medical student at Case Western Reserve University, provided us with splendid assistance from the stage of editing first-draft chapters through the submission of the final manuscript. Marcia Bram provided the high-quality and loyal secretarial assistance that is essential to projects of this nature.

Martha and Jenny Binstock and Mitsuko and Emma Post were very supportive in understanding the priorities and values that engaged us in this undertaking.

Contributors

Robert H. Binstock, Ph.D., is the Henry R. Luce Professor of Aging, Health, and Society at Case Western Reserve University School of Medicine, Cleveland, Ohio. A former president of the Gerontological Society of America (1975–1976), he has served as the director of a White House Task Force on Older Americans (1967–1968) and as chairman and member of many advisory panels to governments and foundations. Binstock is the author of some 100 articles on the politics and the policies affecting aging; the latest of his 16 authored and edited books is *Handbook of Aging and the Social Sciences*, third edition, coedited by Linda George. He is the recipient of many awards in the field of aging.

Christine K. Cassel, M.D., is chief of the Section of General Internal Medicine and professor of medicine and of public policy at the University of Chicago, Chicago, Illinois. She is the author of more than 100 articles in geriatric medicine, medical ethics, and public policy. Her books include *Geriatric Medicine: Principles and Practice* (a two-volume textbook now in its second edition), *Ethical Dimensions in the Health Professions*, and *Nuclear Weapons and Nuclear War: A Source Book for Health Professionals*.

Nancy Neveloff Dubler, L.L.B., is director of the Division of Legal and Ethical Issues in Health Care and associate professor in the Department of Epidemiology and Social Medicine, Montefiore Medical Center/Albert Einstein College of Medicine, New York, New York. She founded and is director of that institution's Ethical Consultation Service. Dubler has served on several advisory committees to the U.S. Congress Office of Technology Assessment, and chairs and serves on a number of other panels and committees dealing with issues of law, ethics, and health. She is the author of numerous articles on these subjects, including many focused on aging. Her books include *Alzheimer's Dementia: Dilemmas in Clinical Research*; *Health Care in Prisons, Jails and Detention Centers: Some Legal and Ethical Dilemmas*; and *Standards for Health Care Services in Correctional Institutions*.

Roger W. Evans, Ph.D., is senior research scientist in the Health and Population Study Center at the Battelle Human Affairs Research Center, Seattle, Washington. He was a member of the National Task Force on Organ Transplantation (1985–1986) and currently serves on the boards of directors of the United Network for Organ Sharing and the National Marrow Donor Program. Evans has written extensively on the clinical and socioeconomic aspects of organ transplantation, the allocation and rationing of health care resources, and the assessment of medical technology.

Dennis W. Jahnigen, M.D., is head of the Section of Geriatric Medicine at the Cleveland Clinic Foundation, Cleveland, Ohio. He has served on the U.S. Surgeon General's Task Force on Preventive Medicine in the Elderly, and on the Needs Assessment Advisory Panel for the Health Care Financing Administration. A participant in the National Institute on Aging's Consensus Panel on Geriatric Assessment in 1987, Jahnigen is on the board of the American Geriatrics Society. His many publications include *Medical Student Source Book for Geriatrics* and a chapter in *Should Medical Care Be Rationed by Age?*.

Harry R. Moody, Ph.D., is deputy director of the Brookdale Center on Aging of Hunter College, New York, New York. He received his doctorate in philosophy from Columbia University. The author of numerous articles, Moody has recently published a book entitled *Abundance of Life: Human Development Policies for an Aging Society*, and he is author of a forthcoming book, *Ethics and Aging*.

Thomas H. Murray, Ph.D., is professor and director of the Center for Biomedical Ethics of Case Western Reserve University School of Medicine, Cleveland, Ohio. He is an elected fellow of the Hastings Center, chair of the Faculty Association of the Society for Health and Human Values, and a founding editor of *Medical Humanities Review*. The author of more than 100 books and articles, Murray writes about a wide range of issues in bioethics and social policy.

Bernice L. Neugarten, Ph.D., is the Rothschild Distinguished Scholar at the Center on Aging, Health, and Society of the University of Chicago, Chicago, Illinois. A former president of the Gerontological Society of America (1969), she is a fellow of the American Academy of Arts and Sciences and a member of the Institute of Medicine, National Academy of Sciences, and was deputy chair for the White House Conference on Aging of 1981. Neugarten is the author of some 160 articles in the field of human development and aging. Her eight books include *Age or Need? Public Policies for Older People*; *Middle Age and Aging*; and *Personality in Middle and Old Age*. She is the recipient of numerous national and international awards in the field of aging.

Stephen G. Post, Ph.D., is assistant professor of biomedical ethics at Case Western Reserve University School of Medicine, Cleveland, Ohio. He is chair of the American Academy of Religion's Group on Religion, Medicine, and Health, and research fellow with the Joseph and Rose Kennedy Institute of Ethics at Georgetown University, Washington, D.C. Post is associate editor of *Encyclopedia of Bioethics*, second edition, and is on the editorial board of *Journal of Medicine Humanities*. A former core research member of the Hastings Center's project on imperiled newborns. Post has published articles in such journals as *Hastings Center Report*, the *Christian Century*, *Journal of the American Geriatrics Society*, the *Gerontologist*, and *Ageing and Society*.

Charles P. Sabatino, J.D., is assistant director of the American Bar Association's Commission on Legal Problems of the Elderly and is adjunct professor of law at Georgetown University Law Center, Washington, D.C. He previously managed a legal services program for elderly people in northern Virginia.

David C. Thomasma, Ph.D., is the Michael I. English Professor of Medical Ethics and director of the Medical Humanities Program at Loyola University's Stritch School of Medicine, Chicago, Illinois, and also chief of the Ethics Consult Service there. He is editor-in-chief of *Theoretical Medicine* and section editor of the *Journal of the American Geriatrics Society*, and is on the editorial boards of four other journals in the field. Thomasma is a member of the Technical Advisory Panel for Biomedical Ethics for the American Hospital Association, and the Theology and Ethics Advisory Committee for the Catholic Health Association. His most recent books are *Medical Ethics: A Guide for Health Professionals*; *For the Patient's Good: Towards the Restoration of Beneficience in Health Care*; and *Theory and Practice in Medical Ethics*. He has written five other books and more than 160 articles.

Too Old for Health Care?

1

Old Age and the Rationing of Health Care

ROBERT H. BINSTOCK, Ph.D., and
STEPHEN G. POST, Ph.D.

Suggestions that health care be denied to older persons in the United States began to emerge in the early 1980s. These proposals, which vary in specific content and in the age ranges they use to define "older persons," have been made with increasing frequency in recent years. In part, they appear to be an expression of a larger backlash against an artificially homogenized group labeled "the aged," which has become a scapegoat for a variety of problems in American society during the past decade.

Compassionate Ageism and the "Old-Age Welfare State"

Before the late 1970s, the predominant stereotypes of older Americans were compassionate. Elderly people were seen as poor, frail, socially dependent, objects of discrimination, and above all deserving (Kalish, 1979). For some 40 years—dating from the Social Security Act of 1935—American society accepted the oversimplified notion that all older persons are essentially the same (Neugarten, 1970) and all are in need of governmental assistance.

The American polity implemented this perception by adopting and financing major benefit programs based on age, and tax and price subsidies for which eligibility is not determined by need. Through Social Security, Medicare, the Older Americans Act, special tax privileges for being aged 65 or older, and a variety of other measures, elderly persons were exempted from the screenings that are applied to other Americans to determine whether they are worthy of public help.

1

During the 1960s and the 1970s, just about every issue that advocates for the elderly could identify as affecting some subgroup of the elderly population became a governmental responsibility: nutritional, legal, supportive, and leisure services; housing; home repair; energy assistance; transportation; help in getting jobs; protection against being fired from jobs; special mental health programs; a separate National Institute on Aging; and so on (Estes, 1979; Kutza, 1981). In the mid-1970s the U.S. House of Representatives, Select Committee on Aging (1976), using loose criteria, was able to identify 134 programs benefiting aging persons, overseen by 49 committees and subcommittees of Congress.

In short, by the late 1970s, if not earlier, American society had learned the catechism of compassionate ageism very well and had expressed it through a variety of governmental programs and objectives that created a "welfare state for the elderly" (Myles, 1989, p. 2). We had rejected proposals for universal national health insurance, for example, but—through Medicare—we were willing to establish national health insurance for elderly people (see Cohen, 1985; Marmor, 1970).

The Emergence of "The Aged" as a Scapegoat

Since 1978, however, the long-standing compassionate stereotypes of older persons have been undergoing an extraordinary reversal (see Binstock, 1983). Older people have come to be portrayed as one of the more flourishing and powerful groups in American society, and have been attacked as a burdensome responsibility. The immediate precipitating factor seems to have been a so-called crisis in the cash flow of the Social Security system, within the larger context of a depressed economy during President Carter's administration (see Estes, 1983).

Two additional elements seem to have contributed importantly to this reversal of stereotypes. One element was a tremendous growth in the amount of federal funds expended on benefits to aging Americans, a phenomenon that journalists (e.g., Samuelson, 1978) and academicians (e.g., Hudson, 1978) began to notice and publicize in the late 1970s. By 1982 an economist in the U.S. Office of Management and Budget had reframed the classical trade-off metaphor of political economy, "guns versus butter," as "guns versus canes" (Torrey, 1982). Throughout the 1980s, about 26 percent of the annual federal budget was spent on benefits to aging persons (U.S. Senate, Special Committee on Aging, 1988).

A second element in the reversal of the stereotypes of old age has been dramatic improvements in the aggregate status of older Americans, in large measure due to the impact of federal benefit programs. Social

Security, for example, has helped to reduce the proportion of elderly persons in poverty from about 35 percent three decades ago (Clark, 1990) to 12.8 percent today (U.S. Senate, Special Committee on Aging, 1988). The success of such programs has improved the average economic status of aged persons to the point where journalists can now accurately depict older Americans as "more prosperous than the general population" (Tolchin, 1988, p. 1).

Regardless of the specific causes, the reversal of stereotypes has continued throughout the 1980s, to the point where we now find—in the media, political speeches, public policy studies, and the writings of scholars—a new set of axioms regarding older people:

- They are relatively well-off—not poor, but in great economic shape.
- They are a potent political force because there are so many of them and they all vote in their self-interest; this "senior power" explains why more than one-quarter of the annual federal budget is spent on benefits to elderly persons.
- Because of demographic changes, elderly people are becoming more numerous and politically powerful and will claim even more benefits and substantially larger proportions of the federal budget. They are already costing too much, and in the future they will pose an unsustainable burden for the American economy.

These new stereotypes, devoid of compassion, can be readily observed in popular culture. Typical of contemporary depictions of older persons was a cover story in *Time* entitled "Grays on the Go" (Gibbs, 1988). It was filled with pictures of senior surfers, senior swingers, and senior softball players. Older persons were portrayed as America's new elite: healthy, wealthy, powerful, and "staging history's biggest retirement party" (p. 66).

A dominant theme in such accounts of older persons is that their selfishness is ruining the nation. The *New Republic* highlighted this motif early in 1988 with a drawing on the cover caricaturing older persons, with the caption "greedy geezers." The table-of-contents "teaser" for the story that followed (Fairlie, 1988) announced that "the real me generation isn't the yuppies, it's America's growing ranks of prosperous elderly." This theme was echoed the following year by a *New York Times* "Opinion-Editorial" headlined "Elderly, Affluent—and Selfish" (Longman, 1989).

In serious forums of public discourse, these new stereotypes of elderly persons as prosperous, hedonistic, and selfish have established a climate of opinion in which the aged have emerged as a scapegoat for an impressive list of American problems. As social psychologist Gordon Allport observed in his classic work *ABC's of Scapegoating*, "An issue seems nicely simplified if we blame a group or class of people rather than the complex course of social and historical forces" (1959, pp. 13–14).

Demographers (e.g., Preston, 1984) and advocates for children have blamed the political power of elderly Americans for the plight of young-sters who have inadequate nutrition, health care, and education, and insufficiently supportive family environments. One children's advocate even proposed that parents receive an "extra vote" for each of their young children, in order to combat older voters (Carballo, 1981). For-mer Secretary of Commerce Peter Peterson (1987) has suggested that, in order for the United States to regain its stature as a first-class power in the world economy, it must make a sharp reduction in programs benefiting older citizens.

A ludicrous manifestation of this trend emerged in 1989, when a distinguished "Executive Panel" of American leaders convened by the Ford Foundation designated older people as the only group of citizens responsible for financing a broad range of social programs for persons of all ages, including infants. In a report entitled *The Common Good: Social Welfare and the American Future*, the panel recommended a series of policies costing a total of $29 billion. How did the panel propose that this $29 billion be financed? Solely by taxation of Social Security benefits (Ford Foundation, 1989, p. 81). In fact, every financing alter-native considered in the report was one that made elderly people the financiers of the panel's package of recommendations for improving everyone's social welfare.

Old-Age-Based Rationing of Health Care

Perhaps the most serious scapegoating of aged people, in terms of in-creasing the vulnerability of older persons and, maybe, all persons in our society, has been with respect to health care. In the past few years, widespread concern about high rates of inflation in health care costs has been refocused from health care providers, suppliers, administrators, and insurers—the parties responsible for setting the prices of care—to the elderly patients for whom health care is provided.

Americans aged 65 and older, about 12 percent of our population, account for one-third of the nation's annual health care expenditures: over $175 billion in 1988 (U.S. House of Representatives, Select Com-mittee on Aging, 1989, p. 4). Because the elderly population is growing, absolutely and proportionately, health care costs for older persons have been depicted as an unsustainable burden, or as one observer has put it, "a great fiscal black hole" that will absorb an unlimited amount of our national resources (Callahan, 1987, p. 17).

This particular theme of scapegoating the aged for high health care costs has developed to the point that many proposals for old-aged-based rationing of health care have been put forward in recent years; some of them suggest official restrictions on the health care insurance provided for persons aged 65 and older through the federal Medicare program, and others argue, in a more generalized fashion, that our society must set limits to health care for persons of advanced old age. The substantial attention that such proposals have received in serious public forums may be the clearest signal that American public policy toward health care of aging persons is approaching an important crossroads.

To be sure, health care in the United States has long been rationed informally on the basis of the immediate availability of resources and the individual conditions and characteristics of patients. However, proposals for official policies that would deny care categorically, on the basis of membership in a demographically identified group, are a substantial departure from existing practices and philosophies.

The suggestion that health care should be rationed on the basis of old age began to develop, through implication, in 1983. In a speech to the Health Insurance Association of America, economist Alan Greenspan, now chairman of the Federal Reserve Board, stated that 30 percent of Medicare funds are annually expended on the 5 to 6 percent of Medicare insurees who die within the year. He pointedly asked "whether it is worth it" (Schulte, 1983, p. 1).

In 1984 Richard Lamm, then governor of Colorado, was widely quoted as stating that older persons "have a duty to die and get out of the way" (Slater, 1984, p. 1). Although Lamm subsequently stated that he had been misquoted on this specific statement, he has been delivering the same message repeatedly since leaving office, in only somewhat more delicately worded fashion (e.g., Lamm, 1987; Lamm 1989a; Lamm 1989b).

During the past few years, discussion of this issue has spread to a number of forums. Philosophers (e.g., Daniels, 1988) have been generating principles of equity to undergird justice between age groups in the provision of health care, rather than, for instance, justice between rich and poor (see Binstock, 1985). Conferences and books with titles such as *Should Medical Care Be Rationed by Age?* (Smeeding et al., 1987) have explicitly addressed the issue.

Late in 1987 this issue received substantial popular attention with the publication of a book entitled *Setting Limits: Medical Goals in an Aging Society*, by a biomedical ethicist, Daniel Callahan (1987). It depicts the elderly population as "a new social threat" and a "demographic, economic and medical avalanche, one that could ultimately (and perhaps already) do [sic] great harm" (p. 20). Callahan's remedy for this threat is to use "age as a specific criterion for the allocation and limitation of health care" (p. 23), by denying life-extending health care, as a matter of public policy, to persons who are aged in their "late 70s or early 80s" and/or have "lived out a natural life span" (p. 171). What is a "natural life span"? Callahan tries to suggest that it is possible to answer this question. According to his vague definition, the natural life span is a matter of biography rather than biology. He uses chronological age as an arbitrary marker to designate when, from a biographical standpoint, the individual should have reached the end of a "natural" life.

Setting Limits received a great deal of national attention. It was reviewed in national magazines, the *New York Times*, the *Washington Post*, the *Wall Street Journal*, and just about every relevant professional and scholarly journal and newsletter. Callahan himself has continued to present and defend his point of view in a subsequent book (Callahan, 1990), and in a number of public forums throughout the country. It appears that proposals for age-based rationing have come to be rather firmly embedded in public discourse about health care policies in the United States.

"Too Old" for Health Care?

The chapters in this present volume are animated by the collective belief of the contributors that proposals for age-based rationing involve many grave issues—some explicit, others implicit—that must aired and thoroughly understood by Americans. Many contemporary discussions of rationing, why it should be undertaken, and how it might be done are cluttered with misunderstandings. Some of the problems that proponents of rationing think that they would solve are, in fact, illusory. Moreover, constructive steps can be taken to meet the geuine health care challenges of an aging society, steps that do not require official policies that would label millions of Americans as "too old" for health care.

Health Care, Health Care Costs, and the Goals of Medicine

One of the persistent themes that appear in proposals for age-based rationing is the assertion that costly, futile, and therefore wasteful efforts are often made to keep older patients alive through the use of expensive, technology-intensive medical interventions, against the patients' wishes. However, in chapter 2, below, Jahnigen and Binstock show that, in fact, most expenditures are not for high-technology interventions. Sketching out the larger context of ever-increasing American health care expenditures and cost-containment concerns, they present the costs of health care for older persons, the sources of payment for those costs, and the distribution of expenditures among various kinds of health care: dramatic technological interventions, physicians, hospitals, nursing homes, home care, and a range of other health services. Then, hypothetically putting aside ethical considerations, they argue that age-based rationing would accomplish very little in terms of cost reduction.

A recurring assumption in discussions of rationing is that patients of advanced age are poor candidates for complicated medical interventions, that is, that they do not derive as much benefit from many treatments as younger adults do. However, Jahnigen and Binstock review the evidence on the factors that predict successful outcomes for a wide variety of medical interventions, and show that old age, in itself, is not a good predictor of success or failure. The important predictors are the patient's underlying clinical condition(s) and his or her functional status.

Roger Evans extends this analysis in chapter 3, with particular attention to life-saving intervention through advanced medical technologies, such as those used in kidney dialysis, liver transplantation, and heart transplantation. So far, the use of these technologies with patients who are in their late seventies and eighties has been rare. However, growing experience with their use in patients who are in their sixties and late fifties shows that persons in this intermediate age range who are selected for such procedures unquestionably benefit from them, sometimes more than younger patients. In addition, some advanced procedures, such as organ transplantation, can be shown to be cost-effective when undertaken with such older patients.

In chapter 4, Christine Cassel and Bernice Neugarten distinguish between the caricature of "heroic" medical interventions undertaken to prolong life, and the technology-intensive efforts that are often undertaken to improve the quality of a patient's life, and may also have the side-effect of prolonging life. The boundary between caring and healing, on the one hand, and prolonging life, on the other hand, is highly permeable in the practice of medicine.

Another theme that recurs in discussions of age-based rationing is the continuing growth of our older population, and the implications of that growth for great increases in future health care demands and expenditures. Our elderly population is not only increasing in size but also growing older on average. As summarized in the Appendix to chapter 3, persons of advanced old age, at present, have substantially higher rates of illness and disability than do persons in their mid-sixties and their seventies. The large future cohorts of persons in their late seventies and their eighties, and older are also likely to experience such comparatively higher rates of morbidity, and thereby to require greater quantities of health care, involving correspondingly greater costs, in the decades immediately ahead.

Jahnigen and Binstock, as well as Cassel and Neugarten, portray various dimensions of this geriatric challenge. Jahnigen and Binstock set forth a "geriatric-sensitive" model of medical practice which puts much greater emphasis on the individual patient's values and nonmedical situations than does the traditional, biomedically oriented model of American medicine. Through this approach, they suggest, many unfortunate instances of inappropriate, painful, and/or needlessly costly treatment of older persons an be avoided. Cassel and Neugarten assess the appropriate goals of medicine in an aging society, and suggest the dimensions of a model of health care practice that is responsive to those goals. Their proposed model attempts to combine the best elements of the more traditional models of medicine—the heroic and the humanistic—by embracing the aging society.

Health Care Rationing and the Law

If old-age rationing were to be widely imposed in the United States, by budgetary or other official means, a highly predictable response would be a flood of litigation attempting to counteract denials of health care. When Aaron and Schwartz studied rationing as it takes place through the British National Health Service, and tried to anticipate the consequences if such practices became prevalent in the United States, they asserted:

> Because of the characteristics of the U.S. tort system, we anticipate that individual and class action suits would be brought by, and on behalf of, many patients denied some potentially beneficial therapy. Suits would be further stimulated if budget limits prevented physicians from making use of the power . . . to sustain the lives of those whose defects are irremediable, and to carry out procedures that defer or repair the consequences of aging. (1984, p. 132)

In chapter 5, Nancy Neveloff Dubler and Charles Sabatino address the issue of whether policies denying life-sustaining care might be legal or illegal under U.S. law. They explore the general status of older persons in the American legal system, under the common law, federal and state legislation, and the U.S. Constitution; and after reviewing the legal rights of older persons to obtain health care, they consider the possible recourses an older person might have if some old-age-based rationing policies were imposed.

Humanistic Perspectives on Rationing

Even as proposals for age-based rationing raise legal questions regarding the basic human rights of older persons, they also evoke issues that require a response from the wider historical tradition of Western humanistic thought. Are these rationing proposals consistent with Jewish and Christian moral values? Religious traditions aside, are such proposals philosophically reasonable? Do they emerge from failure to appreciate the forms of human fulfillment that give meaning to growing old?

Basic to both Jewish and Christian moral thought is the norm of human equality. Human beings are all considered worthy of a fundamental respect regardless of age, race, gender, or social contribution. Moreover, both Judaism and Christianity are deeply suspicious of the human greed and will to power that underlie the perennial temptation to treat some more equally than others. If official health care rationing were ever to become truly necessary, these religious traditions would countenance only those proposals that treated all human beings equally, regardless of age. Stephen Post explicates these dimensions of Jewish and Christian thought in chapter 6 and highlights the reasoning that underlies them.

Religious traditions aside, are age-based rationing proposals consistent with the harmonies and mutualities that allow societies to prosper? Post (in chapter 6) and philosopher David Thomasma (in chapter 7) think not. Both contend that our society can mobilize its energies in creative, positive ways to care for older persons in need so as to enhance intergenerational reciprocities. Ethicist Thomas Murray (in chapter 8) expresses his belief that such reciprocity is discouraged by the negative stereotypes and labels that are attached to elderly people. In contrast to such stereotypes, he examines the forms of meaning that older persons find in the fullness of their years. A common theme to these three chapters—from the perspectives of religious studies, philosophy, literature, and humanistic psychology—is the importance of avoiding proposals likely to result in an adversarial attitude toward elderly people.

What of the ethical principle of respect for autonomy or self-determination? Murray suggests that an official policy mandating age-based rationing would be regarded as so arbitrary and coercive in our contemporary society that it would incite civil disobedience. Thomasma concurs, and argues that instead of rationing, society should require persons to complete living wills or other forms of "advance directives" upon reaching the age of 65. Post emphasizes that few, if any, older persons wish to have their lives prolonged through futile interventions when death is imminent and the quality of life is low.

Those who propose age-based rationing, Thomasma notes, do not fully appreciate the wisdom of the individual elderly person in deciding about appropriate levels of medical intervention. No advocate of rationing has truly explained why coercive methods are necessary, and why older persons cannot make wise choices autonomously. Perhaps an unspoken assumption underlying some rationing proposals is an ageist one, namely, that old persons, because they are old, cannot make good decisions.

The ideas introduced in proposals for rationing may be provocative and stimulating but not necessarily useful. Harry Moody, in chapter 9, acknowledges that the idea of a "natural life course," as discussed by Callahan (1987; 1990), Daniels (1988), and others, is a plausible and stimulating concept when articulated in the abstract. However, he also observes that advocates of age-based rationing have given scant attention, if any, to the question of how their philosophical perspectives could be put into practice.

Advocates of rationing provide startling perspectives, with little concern for translating those perspectives into practicable schemes and examining the issues that would be raised by such schemes. In contrast, Moody explores many examples of how such allocative arrangements already operate in our lives, and provides some feeling for what might be the implications if more such arrangements were instituted to control the allocation of health care. His illustrations, and the suggestions for individual autonomy put forward by Thomasma, suggest a variety of ways in which we might follow Thomas Murray's observation that Americans should decide for ourselves just what a "natural life course" is, and whether any of us is "too old" for health care.

References

Aaron, H.J., and Schwartz, W.B. (1984). *The painful prescription: rationing hospital care*. Washington, D.C.: Brookings Institution.

Allport, G.W. (1959). *ABC's of scapegoating*. New York: Anti-Defamation League of B'nai B'rith.

Binstock, R.H. (1983). The aged as scapegoat. *Gerontologist, 23*, 136–143.

Binstock, R.H. (1985). The oldest-old: a fresh perspective or compassionate ageism revisited? *Milbank Memorial Fund Quarterly/Health and Society, 63*, 420–451.

Callahan, D. (1987). *Setting limits: medical goals for an aging society*. New York: Simon & Schuster.

Callahan, D. (1990). *What kind of life: the limits of medical progress*. New York: Simon & Schuster.

Carballo, M. (1981). Extra votes for parents? *Boston Globe*, December 17, p. 35.

Clark, R.L. (1990). Income maintenance policies in the United States. In R.H. Binstock and L.K. George, eds., *Handbook of aging and the social sciences* (3rd ed.), pp. 382–397. San Diego: Academic Press.

Cohen, W.J. (1985). Reflections on the enactment of Medicare and Medicaid. *Health Care Financing Review*, annual suppl., pp. 3–11.

Daniels, N. (1988). *Am I my parents' keeper? an essay on justice between the young and the old*. New York: Oxford University Press.

Estes, C.L. (1979). *The aging enterprise*. San Francisco: Jossey-Bass.

Estes, C.L. (1983). Social Security: the social construction of a crisis. *Milbank Memorial Fund Quarterly/Health and Society*, 61, 445–461.

Fairlie, H. (1988). Talkin' 'bout my generation. *New Republic*, 198(13), 19–22.

Ford Foundation, Project on Social Welfare and the American Future, Executive Panel (1989). *The common good: social welfare and the American future*. New York: Ford Foundation.

Gibbs, N.R. (1988). Grays on the go. *Time*, 131(8), 66–75.

Hudson, R.H. (1978). The "graying" of the federal budget and its consequences for old age policy. *Gerontologist*, 18, 428–440.

Kalish, R.A. (1979). The new ageism and the failure models: a polemic. *Gerontologist*, 19, 398–407.

Kutza, E.A. (1981). *The benefits of old age*. Chicago: University of Chicago Press.

Lamm, R.D. (1987). A debate: Medicare in 2020. In *Medicare reform and the Baby Boom generation*, edited proceedings of the second annual conference of Americans for Generational Equity, April 30–May 1, 1987, pp. 77–88. Washington, D.C.: Americans for Generational Equity.

Lamm, R.D. (1989a). Columbus and Copernicus: new wine in old wineskins. *Mount Sinai Journal of Medicine*, 56(1), 1–10.

Lamm, R.D. (1989b). Saving a few, sacrificing many—at great cost. *New York Times*, August 8, p. 23.

Longman, P. (1989). Elderly, affluent—and selfish. *New York Times*, October 10, p. 27.

Marmor, T.R. (1970). *The politics of Medicare*. London: Routledge & Kegan Paul.

Myles, J.F. (1989). *Old age in the welfare state: the political economy of public pensions*. Lawrence: University Press of Kansas.

Neugarten, B.L. (1970). The old and the young in modern societies. *American Behavioral Scientist*, 15, 13–24.

Peterson, P. (1987). The morning after. *Atlantic*, 260(4), 43–69.

Preston, S.H. (1984). Children and the elderly in the U.S. *Scientific American*, 251(6), 44–49.

Samuelson, R.J. (1978). Aging America: who will shoulder the growing burden? *National Journal*, 10, 1712–1717.

Schulte, J. (1983). Terminal patients deplete Medicare, Greenspan says. *Dallas Morning News*, April 26, p.1.

Slater, W. (1984). Latest Lamm remark angers the elderly. *Arizona Daily Star*, March 29, p. 1.

Smeeding, T.M., Battin, M.P., Francis, L.P., and Landesman, B.M., eds. (1987). *Should medical care be rationed by age?* Totowa, N.J.: Rowman & Littlefield.

Tolchin, M. (1988). New health insurance plan provokes outcry over costs. *New York Times*, November 2, p. 1.

Torrey, B.B. (1982). Guns vs. canes: the fiscal implications of an aging population. *American Economics Association Papers and Proceedings*, 72, 309–313.

U.S. House of Representatives, Select Committee on Aging (1976). *Federal responsibility to the elderly: executive programs and legislative jurisdiction.* Washington, D.C.: U.S. Government Printing Office.

U.S. House of Representatives, Select Committee on Aging (1989). *Health care costs for America's elderly, 1977–88.* Washington, D.C.: U.S. Government Printing Office.

U.S. Senate, Special Committee on Aging (1988). *Developments in aging: 1987*, vol. 1. Washington: U.S. Government Printing Office.

2

Economic and Clinical Realities: Health Care for Elderly People

DENNIS W. JAHNIGEN, M.D., and
ROBERT H. BINSTOCK, Ph.D.

Many contemporary discussions about the rationing of health care on the basis of old age are laden with misperceptions of what is actually happening in the world of health care for older Americans. The significance of frequently quoted statistics concerning health care costs is often misunderstood, or is not examined. The decision processes by which American physicians actually decide whether and how to treat elderly patients are not widely known.

Health care professionals in this country function within a large and complex $600-billion industry that shapes their behavior. In recent decades physicians' capacity to control American medicine has eroded (see Starr, 1982), and they are influenced much more than in the past by hospital, nursing home, and out-patient markets; decisions by the administrators of health care corporations; private and public insurance reimbursement practices; the development and marketing of new medical technologies; increased litigation regarding medical practice; and governmental policies controlling fees and treatment choices. These economic incentives and constraints of the health care industry, however, tend to obscure the details of how physicians conduct their medical practices and deal with individual patients.

This chapter looks at some of the day-to-day realities in the world of health care for elderly patients. Within the context of an increasingly costly and multifaceted American health care system, it examines the ways in which dollars are actually expended on care for older persons, the health care implications of an increasingly older population, the practices through which American medicine considers and decides on

13

the treatment of elderly patients, and the practical implications of suggestions that health care be rationed on the basis of old age. It also outlines a "geriatric-sensitive" model of medical practice which is a departure from the traditional medical model, and which can improve the appropriateness of decisions regarding the treatment of elderly patients. Finally, it suggests that discussions of justice in the arena of health care are more appropriately and usefully focused upon inequities in the treatment of rich and poor than upon possible inequities in the treatment of old and young.

The Larger Context of Health Care "Cost Containment"

Much of the recent public discourse about health care rationing has been explicitly linked to concerns about rising health care costs. These concerns flared up in the United States during the 1980s in the form of a "cost-containment fever" that shows no sign of subsiding. Since 1950, total consumer health care costs, adjusted for inflation, have risen at an annual rate of 5.5 percent (Aaron and Schwartz, 1990). By 1987 the nation's annual health care expenditure had exceeded $500 billion and was more than 11 percent of the gross national product (GNP), nearly double the proportion of the GNP that it had been in 1965 when Medicare, the national health insurance program for persons aged 65 and older, was enacted by Congress (Letsch et al., 1988).

At the outset of the 1980s, the governmental and corporate entities that pay for an overwhelming proportion of American health care began attempting to limit their financial obligations (Thurow, 1985). California, Massachusetts, and several other states enacted statutes—at the behest of insurance companies and large corporate employers—to curb hospital costs (Kinzer, 1983). In 1983 the federal government limited Medicare reimbursements to hospitals by implementing a "prospective payment system" through which the amounts reimbursed for each Medicare inpatient were fixed in accordance with a "diagnosis-related-group" (DRG) classification rather than the length of the hospital stay and the services received by the patient (Latta and Helbing, 1988). By the end of the decade, executives of major corporations were breaking a long-standing taboo by announcing their support for the notion of national health insurance, as a means of cutting their firms' costs for employees' health insurance premiums and redistributing the expense to U.S. taxpayers (see Freudenheim, 1989a; Freudenheim, 1989c).

Health Care Costs: How Much Is "Too Much"?

As this movement toward cost containment has developed, it has been accompanied by a chorus of claims that we are spending "too much" of our national resources on health care (e.g., Lamm, 1989). Health policy analysts who want us to curb our national health care investment feel that larger expenditures for health care will have adverse consequences for American economic competitiveness, government budgets, and a variety of other social and economic responsibilities (see Mechanic, 1985a).

Although health care cost containment is a reasonable political objective, it is not mandated by any "iron law" of economics. Advocates of cost containment warn that we cannot sustain increasing health care expenditures, but they do not spell out the inevitable dire consequences that would ensue for our nation if such expenditures continue to increase. It is not at all clear that escalating health care costs hurt the global position of the American economy. Despite the current laments about the economic decline of the United States, our share of the world GNP has held constant at 23 percent since the mid-1970s (Nye, 1990), a period during which our health care costs have increased annually at a rate ranging from two to three times our general rate of inflation. As many qualified observers have pointed out (e.g., Schwartz and Aaron, 1985), there is no inherent reason why 11 to 13 percent, or more, of our GNP can not be expended on health care.

It is true, of course, that the more we spend on health care, the less we have for other goods, services, and purposes. But this is a genuine choice. Among the industrialized nations of the world, the United States has chosen to be the "odd man out" in its approaches to financing and providing health care (Abel-Smith, 1985, p. 16). Although most of us probably would like to eliminate wasteful expenditures, we may continue to prefer our basic approaches to health care, even at the expense of other goods and services.

Comparisons with other countries provide a political frame of reference for arguing that the United States spends too much. We do spend far more of our national wealth on health care than any other developed nation does. For instance, the proportion of U.S. resources allocated to health care expenditures is 74 percent greater than the corresponding figure for the United Kingdom and 27 percent greater than the share expended on health care in Canada (Waldo et al., 1986). On the other hand, Americans might not be satisfied with the levels of care generally available in these or other nations. The quality of health care provided as a result of the smaller proportions of national wealth spent on it in the United Kingdom, Canada, and elsewhere has been increasingly questioned by both indigenous and foreign observers of those systems.

Both the British and Canadian systems, for example, are predominantly public and are characterized by universal access to care within the context of fixed, governmentally financed budgets. Among the problems that have been noted in the public sectors of these less-expensive systems are the use of old age and other demographic characteristics in Britain to deny care, such as life-saving treatment for kidney failure; long waiting lists for diagnostic tests and for elective surgery, such as hip replacement; back-ups of patients in emergency rooms; shortages of physicians and sophisticated technology; and, with all this, overspent health care budgets (on the United Kingdom, see Aaron and Schwartz, 1984; Aaron and Schwartz, 1990; Grimes, 1987; and Smith, 1989; on Canada, see Barber, 1989; Freudenheim, 1989b; Iglehart, 1986; Lerner, 1990; Walker, 1989). Prime Minister Thatcher has proposed a reorganization of the British health care system in response to such complaints about the quality of care, but her proposal presupposes that the level of expenditures will remain constant. Reportedly, the British Medical Association views the new plan as one that will engender a competition of "the health of the patient versus the cost of the treatment" (Whitney, 1989).

As such comparisons indicate, there are no universal or scientific criteria for determining how much is too much for a nation to spend on health care. The proportion of our national wealth that we can or ought to invest in health care is, of course, a value judgment that will be resolved through politics.

Cost Containment and Rationing

Regardless of competing value judgments as to the appropriate fraction of the GNP to spend on health care, cost containment appears to have become an end in itself in the United States. As it has, widespread concern has been expressed, in professional and public forums, that we will need to ration health care on a scale far greater than ever before, and will need to do so through public policy (see Aaron and Schwartz, 1990).

In fact, in 1989 Alameda County, California, and the state of Oregon became the first governments in the nation to begin a process of explicitly rationing health care among patients in their jurisdictions who are covered by Medicaid, the federal-state health insurance program for the medically indigent (Garland, 1989; Gross, 1989). In order to establish expenditure priorities for staying within their Medicaid budgets, both governments drew up lists ranking medical procedures on the basis of age and sex categories, as well as health care need. In the Oregon list, for instance, some highly ranked services are family planning, prenatal care, preventive dentistry for children, and routine dental care for the elderly; lower rankings are given to foot care for the elderly, eye and hearing exams for nonelderly adults, education of teenagers regarding drug abuse, and organ transplantation. If this plan is approved by the federal government, the state intends to cover only those services ranked most highly, as a means of staying within its budget.

Rationing, of course, is not a new phenomenon in American health care. It has long taken place informally in the context of emergency room "triage," or longer-term waiting-list situations in which only so many health care personnel or so much medication, equipment, or space may be available (Blank, 1988). Health care resources are also allocated unequally on the basis of social class and the ability to pay (Churchill, 1987). Although the creation of Medicare and Medicaid in 1965 increased the equality of access to health care among Americans, it is still evident that many procedures, even relatively low-cost ones, such as immunization, are not readily available to persons of low economic and social status (Hiatt, 1987).

The Costs of Health Care for Older Americans

As indicated in chapter 1 of this book, much of the contemporary cost-containment dialogue has been focused on setting limits to the health care provided to older persons. This tendency to focus on rationing the care of older persons cannot be attributed simply to widespread gerontophobia (dislike or fear of older persons). Indeed, later chapters in this book make it clear that the cultural, religious, and philosophical traditions that have been integral to the development of American society explicitly affirm the worth of older persons. Economic explanations may be more plausible.

First, we currently spend a substantial proportion of our national health care dollars on older Americans, and even larger amounts will be needed in the future. Persons aged 65 and older account for one-third of the annual health care expenditures in the United States—over $175 billion in 1988 (U.S. House of Representatives, Select Committee on Aging, 1989). Simple extrapolations from this present expenditure pattern and from the projected future growth in the number and proportion of older persons in the population imply enormous growth in the amount and the percentage of our national health care expenditures that will be devoted to health care for aging persons in the decades ahead (Committee on an Aging Society, 1985).

Second, Medicare, which insures almost all Americans aged 65 and older, tends to focus cost-containment attention on those who are elderly. The Medicare program, widely perceived as "the health program for the elderly" (although some 3 million other persons, about one-tenth of Medicare insurees, are eligible for the program because they are permanently disabled or have end-stage kidney disease), is the biggest single source of payment for health care in the United States (Health

Care Financing Administration, 1987). Because it is a federal program, its large aggregate national costs are easily determined and become readily visible. In 1987, for example, Medicare paid $81 billion for health care for the elderly and others (Letsch et al., 1988). Moreover, changes in Medicare's approach to paying for care are a plausible strategy for implementing the more general goal of cost containment, since this nationwide governmental program affects the financial incentives of a very high percentage of American hospitals, nursing homes, physicians, and other health care providers and suppliers. In fact, the most widely publicized and far-reaching cost-containment measures to date have been the changes in reimbursement procedures under Medicare's implementation of DRGs.

Who Pays the Costs?

Although Medicare is often perceived as "universal health insurance for the elderly," it only pays 40 percent of older persons' health care costs (U.S. House of Representatives, Select Committee on Aging, 1989, p. 4). Another 18 percent is paid for by other government programs, including Medicaid.

Older persons themselves finance just under 42 percent of their aggregate care. They pay 29 percent in direct out-of-pocket expenditures and pay an additional 4 percent in Medicare premiums and 8 percent in private insurance premiums. These payments by older persons, like health care payments generally, have inflated substantially in recent years—more than tripling, for example, between 1977 and 1988. Perhaps of greater concern to older persons with limited or moderate incomes is the growth of out-of-pocket costs, from under 13 percent of income to over 18 percent of income for the average elderly household during the same period (U.S. House of Representatives, Select Committee on Aging, 1989, p. 8).

Where Do the Health Care Dollars Go?

The use and the costs of technology-intensive medicine are a central focus in most current discussions of whether American society should deny or limit health care to older persons (e.g., Callahan, 1987; Daniels, 1988; U.S. Congress, Office of Technology Assessment, 1987). For some years the press has provided dramatic accounts of organ transplants and other forms of surgery performed on persons in their seventies, eighties, and nineties (e.g., Koenig, 1986), and has reported on the legal issues involving the extended ordeals of older patients who linger on the edge of death in hospitals, sustained only by mechanical ventilators and/or by nutrition obtained through intravenous tube feeding (e.g., Kleiman, 1985).

However, the majority of the funds expended on health care for the aged in the United States are spent neither for hospital care nor for dramatic technological interventions. Only a negligible proportion of elderly nursing-home patients are treated with life-sustaining technologies such as mechanical ventilation, resuscitation, and nutritional support through tube or intravenous feeding (U.S. Congress, Office of Technology Assessment, 1987); nursing homes account for 21 percent of health expenditures on older persons, and cost an average of about $24,000 per year per patient (U.S. Senate, Special Committee on Aging, 1989). A wide range of nonhospital and nonphysician health services (e.g., prescription drugs, dental care, home health care, vision and hearing aids, and medical equipment and supplies) accounts for 16 percent of expenditures; and physicians' fees for outpatient and inpatient services account for 22 percent. The remaining 41 percent comprises payments to hospitals.

Studies in both the United States (Scitovsky, 1984) and Canada (Roos et al., 1987) indicate that aggressive medical interventions are comparable across adult age groups in the last years of life. The greatest difference between younger and older adults with respect to the expenditures associated with dying is that the elderly are far more likely to incur expenses for nursing homes and home care services. In fact, a study of several hundred older persons who died within a 12-month period indicates that severely impaired geriatric patients who received only supportive care, little of which was provided by hospitals and physicians, averaged only slightly smaller expenses for the year (about 8 percent smaller) than did the most expensive decedents who were treated aggressively with technology-intensive measures (Scitovsky, 1988).

The Geriatric Challenge

These contemporary costs are only a small harbinger of the much greater expenditures on health care for older persons which will be required throughout the next several decades. The aggregate population conventionally termed "old" is not only growing but also becoming older, on average, within itself. Among older old-age groups, the rates of disease and disability are much greater than the rates for the total group of persons aged 65 and over. Consequently, as the Institute of Medicine has pointed out, the aging of our older population will present an enormous geriatric challenge to our health care system in the coming decades (Committee on an Aging Society, 1985).

The Elderly Population Is Growing Older

The phenomenon of population aging is now rather well recognized in contemporary society. We have become familiar with the broad outlines of the basic demographic facts and projections. Some 32 million Americans are now aged 65 and older and account for 12.5 percent of our population. The number of persons in this age group is projected to more than double, to 69 million, by the middle of the next century. As early as the year 2030, fully 20 percent of Americans are likely to be aged 65 and over (Taeuber, 1990).

Not so widely understood, however, is the fact that the distribution of age groups within the population aged 65 and older is changing markedly and will continue to do so. In 1980, for example, persons aged 85 and over constituted only 8.8 percent of the American older population; for 1990 they are estimated at 10.3 percent of that group, and in the year 2000 they will be over 13 percent. Similarly, in 1980 persons aged 75 and older constituted 39 percent of the older population; in 1990 they are estimated at 42 percent of it, and by 2000 they will be 48 percent (U.S. Senate, Special Committee on Aging, 1989). Viewed another way, by the end of this century the median person in the 65-plus age group will be just under 75 years of age.

Although the aging of the population has not been a major factor in determining medical care costs in the past (Health Care Financing Administration, 1987, p. 15), this continuous shift toward an increasingly older old-age population has enormous potential implications for geriatric medicine and for expenditures on health care.

Older Old-Age Groups Use More Health Care

Specific older age groupings within the population aged 65 and over use substantially more health care than younger elderly persons do. A few examples readily illustrate this point.

At present, persons aged 65 and older account for 40.5 percent of the days of care in "short-stay" (as opposed to chronic disease) hospitals in the United States. Within that aggregate, those aged 85 and older use hospitals at a rate that is 123 percent higher than that seen among those aged 65 to 74; and persons aged 75 to 84 use hospitals at a rate 69 percent higher than persons aged 65 to 74 (National Center for Health Statistics, 1987c).

Similarly, about 1 percent of Americans aged 65 to 74 years are in nursing homes; this compares with 6 percent of persons 75 to 84 years of age, and 22 percent of persons aged 85 and older (Hing, 1987). The greater numbers of persons who soon will be in the older old-age categories is a major factor in projections that the current nursing-home

Table 2.1
Estimated Percentage of Aged Americans with Functional Limitations Living in the Community, by Age

Age (years)	Percentage
65–69	7.7
70–74	9.7
75–79	13.7
80–85	19.1
≥85	26.6

Source: Gornick et al., 1985, p. 22
Note: *Functional limitations* are defined as limitations in the activities of daily living (e.g., feeding, toileting, bathing, dressing, getting in and out of bed). *Living in the community* is defined as living in a residence other than a hospital, nursing home, or other health care institution in the United States.

population of 1.3 million persons will increase to 2.0 million by the year 2000 and will reach 4.6 million some 40 years later (United States Senate, Special Committee on Aging, 1989).

The same pattern holds true among older persons who, because of functional limitations in their activities of daily living, need home health services from paid professionals or from their families or friends on an in-kind basis. Table 2.1 shows the dramatic increases, by five-year age increments, in the percentage of a contemporary cohort of older persons residing in the community who have limitations in the activities of daily living (e.g., feeding, toileting, bathing, dressing, and getting in and out of bed). The proportion needing help rises from 7.7 percent in the 65- to 69-year-old category to 26.6 percent in the group aged 85 and over, with the largest percentage increase occurring between the 70- to 74-year-old and 75- to 79-year-old categories.

As suggested by these comparisons among older groups, the age-specific prevalence of many acute and long-term chronic diseases and other disabling conditions rises exponentially among populations in their late seventies and in their eighties (Manton, 1990). It is possible, of course, that advances could be made in preventing and treating urinary incontinence, osteoporosis, stroke, dementia, and other geriatric conditions. Recent reports of successful clinical trials in treating osteoporosis in women (Watts et al., 1990) and in promoting the growth of bone mass and lean body mass in older men (Rudman et al., 1990), for example, provide some hints of a basis for long-run optimism. Major breakthroughs would have substantial impact in delaying the onset of chronic illness and disability to older ages than at present, thereby reducing both the prevalance and the duration of illness near the end of the life span, and the health care it requires. A few biomedical researchers and physicians have written optimistically about the possibility of such a "compression of morbidity" at the end of life, painting a scenario in which we are all relatively healthy until shortly before we die (Fries, 1987). To date, unfortunately, there is no scientific evidence to support such an optimistic paradigm (Schneider and Guralnik, 1987).

One can be relatively confident that treatment and prevention modalities will improve and that the organization, financing, and delivery mechanisms of health care will continue to change in the years ahead. However, comparisons among older age groups with respect to their present hospital and nursing home utilization rates suggest that no matter how the terrain of the health care arena evolves in the years ahead, the changing age structure within the older population will, in itself, have a substantial impact on the nature and the volume of the demand for care, and the increased resources necessary to respond to it. A recent projection suggests, for example, that Medicare costs for persons aged 85 and older may increase sixfold by the year 2040, as estimated in constant, inflation-adjusted dollars (Schneider and Guralnik, 1990).

This imminent geriatric challenge, like the current cost of health care for the aging, has certainly played a role in engendering proposals to ration or set limits to health care for older persons. In effect, such proposals call for reforming the customary practices through which American medicine deals with elderly patients. Before examining the practical implications of such proposals for reform through rationing, let us briefly consider the decisions and the medical interventions that American physicians currently employ in treating older patients, and examine what is known about old age as a predictor of the outcome of treatment.

Old Age and the Practice of American Medicine

Many critics view today's physicians as attempting to prolong life at any cost. Elderly persons feel uncertainty about the quality of their relationships with their doctors and express a fear of an impersonal medical care system that may impose upon them unwanted therapies of useless or dubious value (American Medical Association, 1984; Mechanic, 1985b; Okrent, 1987). Some observers attribute this fear to what they term medicine's view of death as an enemy to be defeated (Callahan, 1987; Callahan, 1990). Others see physicians as motivated by greed, refusing despite poor prognoses to let elderly patients who are covered by Medicare die, and yet unwilling to treat needy and uninsured persons. As one prominent critic recently put it, "American medicine grew out of a tradition of professional entrepreneurship, not public service" (Enthoven, 1989, p. 19). Such fears and views are unfortunate for a number of reasons, not the least of which is that they distort and obscure medicine's role in advocating effective medical therapies for older persons.

The Clinical Objectives of Medical Care

As noted at the outset of this chapter, many forces have an impact on the contemporary practice of medicine. Economic incentives and constraints, as well as societal and individual expectations, undoubtedly influence clinical decisions.

Within this larger perspective of health care as an industry, however, it is important to reexamine the clinical objectives of medicine as a caring art. If its fundamental principles are flawed when applied to elderly patients—indeed, patients of any age—contemporary clinical practices must be questioned. If the traditional professional values of medicine are still valid, they can serve as a yardstick for measuring ways in which the practice of medicine may need to change in order to resolve contemporary shortcomings in health care for the elderly.

Traditionally, Western medicine has had three simply stated clinical objectives: to cure where possible, to comfort when appropriate, and to care always.

Historically, all available useful therapies (and some subsequently found to be not so useful) have been employed to achieve these objectives. The search for cures, improved treatment, or palliation of symptoms continues as one of the primary forces behind medical research. When cure is possible it is sought. When cure is not possible, rehabilitation can help in some cases; in other cases the provision of proper care can help to prevent the development of further complicating illnesses. In the cases of hopelessly ill and dying patients, physicians in all eras have recognized the inevitability of death and have used palliative medications and therapies, along with care, to provide comfort and relief of pain (Wanzer et al., 1984). The widespread acceptance of hospice programs in the United States over the last decade has provided an institutional vehicle for undertaking this approach.

In the context of these objectives, old age should be and normally is taken into account in clinical decision making (Barondess et al., 1988). Some factors associated with a decreased likelihood of success in medical interventions do have a relationship with advancing old age, yet for contemporary older Americans, the average life expectancy is not inconsequential. The likelihood of death in the next year for a 65-year-old person is about 3 percent, as compared with about 15 percent for an 85-year-old. A woman aged 65 can expect to live almost 20 years more, and the average woman aged 85 will live over 7 years. A man aged 75 is likely to live almost 10 more years (National Center for Health Statistics, 1987b).

Old Age and Physicians' Decisions

Physicians increasingly are recognizing elderly persons' statistical chances to have substantial periods of extended life, and accordingly, medical intervention practices have become more aggressive with respect to selected older patients. (See chapter 3 for a detailed discussion of the increasing use of advanced medical technology on older patients.) For example, complex surgery is now performed safely, with good results, on some persons in their eighties and nineties (Edmunds et al., 1988; Hosking et al., 1989; Loop et al., 1988). These patients, however, are a carefully selected sample chosen on the basis of their being likely to benefit; they are not a random sample of elderly persons. While physicians may be aggressive in their use of surgery to treat some old persons, they are highly selective in recommending surgery in these cases (see Scitovsky, 1988).

At the same time, studies indicate that physicians also recognize the futility of many interventions for older persons, depending on the patient's disease and level of functioning. In most hospitals and nursing homes, procedures exist (and are used) which permit the withholding of certain types of care (La Puma et al., 1988; Youngner et al., 1985). Patients with advanced dementia are likely to receive comfort measures only and are unlikely to be admitted to an intensive care unit (Miles and Ryder, 1985). In short, although some variability remains in physicians' behavior in such circumstances (Pearlman et al., 1982), many studies suggest that physicians do actively take old age into account in deciding the type and the level of health care services appropriate for their patients (Gillick, 1988).

Such decisions have become much more difficult during the last few decades because life-sustaining technologies have developed very rapidly. These developments have included highly effective methods of artificial feeding, maintenance of circulation, and ventilation; cardiac-assist devices; kidney dialysis; surgical advances in organ transplantation, joint replacement, vascular procedures, and radical cancer surgery. In addition, improvements in the nursing care of comatose or immobile patients can permit the maintenance of skin, bowel, and bladder function for prolonged periods.

These technologies have made dramatic recoveries possible. However, they have also led to situations in which the outcome essentially has been the prolongation of the process of dying. The ready availability of such technology in emergency circumstances, combined with an absence of prior discussions between the physician and the patient (or family) and a lack of satisfactory prognostic information, has all too often contributed to such inappropriate occurrences. However, a number of studies indicate that even when such events occur, physicians do eventually withdraw futile care with the support of family members, and with the backing of ethical and legal precedent (Areen, 1987; Lo, 1980; Ruark et al., 1988). With the increasing use of "living wills" and durable powers of attorney (see chapter 7), which protect physicians who respect patients' wishes for restricted treatment, such withdrawal of futile care will likely be more common in the future.

The development of the highly technical medical specialties necessary for the application of such advanced and complex technologies has also complicated the process of deciding whether aggressive medical intervention is warranted. Medical specialists offer a repertoire of potentially useful interventions; but unless primary care physicians work continuously with them, the specialists often do not possess the full range of information for determining whether an intervention should, in fact, be performed.

Because specialists are involved with a patient only episodically or for a specific procedure, it is often difficult for them to establish the intimacy of the traditional doctor-patient relationship, in which the individual patient's unique personal history, values, wishes, and prognosis can appropriately be taken into account in making decisions. However, when treating an elderly patient, access to highly technical interventions may be essential. Medicine has yet to organize itself so as to optimally combine the skills of the specialist and the primary care physician in the decision-making processes that determine patient care.

Old Age as a Predictor of Clinical Outcomes

As physicians use old age as a factor in their medical decisions, how is it put into play? What kind of weight is it given, in what circumstances?

Advanced age is statistically associated with a reduced likelihood of a favorable outcome for some medical interventions. As a single factor or an independent variable, however, old age is a poor predictor of clinical outcome. The prime reason that old age is a poor single-factor predictor of the outcome of an intervention is that older persons are tremendously diverse, physiologically and psychologically. In fact, the elderly display greater heterogeneity than do younger adults in many measurable aspects of physiologic and psychological function (Fries and Crapo, 1981; Shock et al., 1984).

Heterogeneity among older persons. This phenomenon of heterogeneity among older persons has been observed with regard to many characteristics (Besdine, 1980), and undermines stereotyped assumptions about "normal aging." It also makes predictions about the utility of medical diagnosis and treatment of older persons more difficult.

In general, research on older populations reveals a much wider range between the highest and the lowest measurements of a given function than is seen in studies of younger persons (Rowe, 1977; Rowe and Binstock, 1987; Rowe et al., 1976). Recent research has begun to reveal specific biomedical, behavioral, and socioeconomic predictors of such variations among older persons (Brody, 1989).

Studies of intelligence provide an example of this tendency. Some aspects of measured intelligence decline, on the average, at older ages. However, 15 percent of persons aged 65 and older continue to display progressive intellectual improvement when studied longitudinally (La-bouvie-Vief, 1985). Decline in an older group's average performance over time is not due only to aging. It is in part attributable to the increased prevalence at older ages of diseases that lead to impairment of thinking. Diminished mental ability can be caused, for instance, by primary brain disorders such as Alzheimer's disease and Parkinson's disease or by medical conditions that diminish blood flow to the brain, such as anemia or congestive heart failure. Medications, as well, can have the side effect of diminished mental functioning.

Similarly, the measurement of functional impairments among older persons reflects a tremendous range and diversity. As indicated earlier (see Table 2.1), the percentage of noninstitutionalized persons with limitations in their activities of daily living increases among older subgroups of the elderly population, ranging from 7.7 percent among persons aged 65 through 69 to 26.6 percent among persons aged 85 and older (Gornick et al., 1985). Even in the oldest subgroup, however, the vast majority of persons have no limitations, live independently, and judge their own health to be qualitatively acceptable (National Center for Health Statistics, 1987a).

Old age and other predictors. This heterogeneity among older persons is manifested through substantial variation among them with respect to their potential for benefiting from health care services. Consequently, advanced age, by itself, is an inadequate criterion to use for categorical exclusion from medical diagnosis or intervention.

Even for some technologically sophisticated and aggressive medical interventions, old age does not stand out as a predictor of negative results. Studies of the outcome of in-hospital cardiopulmonary resuscitation (CPR), in general, show survival discharge rates ranging from 1 percent to 20 percent depending upon the population studied (Burns et al., 1989; Gordon and Hurowitz, 1984). The strong predictors of negative outcome are severe preexisting illnesses of certain types (e.g., cancer, stroke, and end-state renal disease); old age is a relatively weak predictor. A study of patients who were resuscitated before they were hospitalized found that 47 percent of the younger patients but only 29 percent of the older patients survived to the time of hospital discharge. The older patients who survived did not stay hospitalized longer, however, and were equivalent to younger patients in neurologic function and in survival after discharge from the hospital (Tresch et al., 1989). When age alone is examined as an independent variable, it is not a very useful predictor of the outcome of the procedure. Far more predictive are such factors as the patient's level of disability and living arrangements, the specific underlying illness present, and the severity of the disease (Bedell et al., 1983). In general, elderly persons who enter the hospital with levels of health and functionality, and with living arrangements, comparable to those of a younger person can expect comparably successful outcomes from CPR efforts.

The intensive care unit is often cited as a high-cost environment where elderly persons receive futile medical care. Here, too, however, when age is viewed as an independent variable, some elderly persons are found to show clear positive outcomes, comparable to those of younger persons, from intensive care (Sage et al., 1987). Moreover, the popular conception that elderly persons are frequently subjected to "Faustian technologies" of intensive care (Lamm, 1989, p. 6), with their own wishes overridden by the urgings of family members, the professional obligations of physicians, and perhaps the fear of malpractice litigation, is wrong. Research indicates that the wishes of elderly patients regarding such care are respected (e.g., Schwartz and Reilly, 1986). In one study of elderly persons who survived intensive care, only 8 percent indicated that they would *not* be willing to return to intensive care units should the need arise (Danis et al., 1988).

Elderly patients can benefit as much or more than younger patients from many other types of health care interventions that are generally considered "aggressive" and of moderately high cost. Surgical procedures such as cataract extraction with intraocular lens implant, or total knee or hip replacement can add immeasurable quality to the life of an older person, with the benefits far outweighing the risks (Blakeslee, 1989).

Some of the more reliable predictors of the utility of medical interventions do have a relationship with age. Perhaps this is why some people are inclined to think that age, at first consideration, would be a suitable criterion for rationing or setting limits on health care.

Life expectancy is one measure that is a superior predictor of the efficacy of medical care. Obviously, advancing age indicates a shorter life expectancy; but the underlying disease and its prognosis are far more important criteria to keep in mind when making decisions on the basis of life expectancy. Consider the case of a 74-year-old man with a cardiac condition, who has been diagnosed as having terminal cancer and is not expected to live more than six months. A medical decision as to whether he could benefit from coronary artery bypass surgery, obviously, would be most heavily weighted by his disease and prognosis, not his age. The concept of *active life expectancy* (Katz et al., 1983), a more refined measure, has been introduced as being potentially more useful for clinical decision making than is life expectancy because it takes into account the patient's likely autonomy and independence, and other qualitative dimensions of his or her remaining life.

Functional status is also a better predictor of the utility of medical care than is age. Functional status is a reflection of the need (or the lack of need) for various levels of assistance in the performance of the activities of daily living. Although older persons are more likely to have impairment of functional status than are younger persons, most elderly persons do not require the physical assistance of others. Although the likelihood of needing nursing home care increases with age, 80 percent of those aged 80 and older live in the community and receive varying degrees of supportive services.

What Could Age-Based Rationing Accomplish?

While American medicine largely has been taking a case-by-case or individualized approach to decisions on the treatment of older patients, suggestions for the categorical rationing of health care for older persons have been put forward to change this. Most of these suggestions, though not all of them (see Callahan, 1987; Callahan, 1990), appear to be motivated by a concern for limiting health care costs. None of them have been very specific as to how rationing on the basis of old age would practicably be undertaken, and what its consequences would be.

For example, Richard Lamm makes clear his view that we cannot afford to spend more on health care for the elderly population, but he does not make clear what steps we should take to limit such expenditures (Lamm, 1987; Lamm, 1989). Daniel Callahan's proposal (1987; 1990) that older persons be denied life-saving care is too vague to be assessed in practical terms. He puts it forward for long-term discussion, and recognizes that "only a full-scale change in habits, thinking, and attitudes would work to make it morally and socially possible" (Callahan, 1987, p. 158). As will be discussed more fully in later chapters, the contributors to the present volume agree that, fortunately, the principle embodied in his proposal—the denial of life-saving care to a demographically defined group—currently is morally and socially unacceptable.

One theme that recurs in the various discussions of old-age-based rationing does lend itself to a limited assessment of its practicability and consequences. It is the repeated lament that a large amount of health care resources is "wasted" by treating patients, particularly Medicare patients, who are in their last 6 to 12 months of life (see Robinson, 1989; Schulte, 1983). Implicitly, if not explicitly, this lament is a proposal to ration the treatment of dying older patients. The economic concept is simple: it is foolish to make investments in projects that will have no return.

Suppose it were possible, both clinically and ethically, to prospectively identify those Medicare patients who were going to die within the year, and whose treatment would be comparatively costly; to choose to not undertake aggressive treatment of them; and thereby to save "unnecessary" health care costs. How much would be saved in terms of Medicare resources and the nation's annual health expenditures? To the extent it is possible to estimate the figure, not very much.

Old Age and the Costs of Dying

The best available data for examing this hypothetical situation are from studies of Medicare expenditures on patients who died and who survived during a 12-month period. There are important limitations to such studies. One weakness is that they do not follow the surviving patients beyond the 12-month period to see exactly how long they survive. Another limitation is that even though some of these studies were published in 1984, the data they examine are from 1979 and earlier. They are the best sources available, however, and—most relevant to the point at issue—well over 90 percent of the patients in the studies were aged 65 and over.

Four Medicare studies analyzed by Scitovsky (1984) all show the same general trends and relationships, although their absolute figures differ slightly. Of the four, the one study most worth examining with respect to the issues raised above is the one by Lubitz and Prihoda (1984), which is the latest, and the most detailed and sophisticated, dealing with Medicare expenditures for the year 1978.

This study and the others substantiate the gist of the public assertions that a high proportion of Medicare funds are expended on persons who are in their last year of life. It found that about 6 percent of Medicare enrollees, those who died within the year, accounted for about 28 percent of Medicare's annual expenditures (Lubitz and Prihoda, 1984). Extrapolated to 1987, when the total Medicare expenditure was

$81 billion (Letsch et al., 1988), this would mean that about $22.7 billion in Medicare funds was used to reimburse health care for the approximately 6 percent of Medicare enrollees who died during the year.

How Costly Are High-Cost Medicare Decedents?

To portray the potential for financial savings, one would want to begin by looking at the high-cost decedents (as opposed to the vast majority, who die shortly after entering the hospital, or die in a nursing home where they do not receive aggressive medical intervention, and thus incur relatively small per capita charges associated with the terminal phase of illness). The Lubitz and Prihoda nationwide study (1984) indicates that a relatively small number and percentage of decedents have comparatively high-cost health care in the last year of life. It found that in 1978 only 3 percent of Medicare-insured decedents had reimbursements of $20,000 or more, and that they accounted for 3.5 percent of total Medicare expenditures that year.

This $20,000 per capita figure for the high-cost Medicare decedents would undoubtedly be much larger today, since health care costs have increased substantially in the ensuing decade (U.S. House of Representatives, Select Committee on Aging, 1989, p. 10). In contemporary terms, what might such per capita expenditures amount to in the aggregate? If potential high-cost decedents could be prospectively identified, and were not treated, what would be the total financial savings?

Extrapolating to a more recent year, the 3.5 percent of Medicare funds spent on high-cost decedents in 1978 would correspond to a total of $2.8 billion for 1987. To be sure, changing medical practices such as the introduction of high-cost technologies and low-cost hospice programs may have had a net effect of increasing or decreasing the percentage of Medicare funds spent on high-cost decedents since 1978. However, even an increase of one or two percentage points would not substantially change the general picture.

In the context of 1987, in which national health care expenditures were $500 billion and Medicare expenditures were $81 billion (Letsch et al., 1988), saving an estimated $2.8 billion would have been useful, but not a matter of overall economic significance. If there is some sort of crisis in health care costs in the United States, saving such an amount, in itself, would have a negligible effect on the overall situation. Nonetheless, some analysts and professionals may feel it is important to conserve such health care resources when their use will not be beneficial. Can it be done?

Can Expenditures for High-Cost Decedents Be Deemed "Wasteful" or "Unnecessary"?

Regardless of the precise amount and the overall economic significance of the dollars that theoretically might be saved by not treating high-cost Medicare decedents, is there any practicable way that such a sum could be saved? Suppose our nation were firmly resolved, as a matter of public policy, to eliminate *all* wasteful and unnecessary health care expenditures. If it were ethically palatable to do so, would it be possible to eliminate such waste by not treating Medicare patients who are likely to be expensive decedents? Only, apparently, if we are willing to withhold treatment from costly patients who will recover—to throw those high-cost patients who would survive into the same "wastebasket" as the costly decedents.

Lubitz and Prihoda (1984) found about the same numbers of survivors and decedents in the high-cost category described above, and almost the same aggregate expenditures on them. Of 49,000 Medicare enrollees in the high-cost category, 25,000 survived and 24,000 died.

If reliable prospective distinctions could be made between high-cost survivors and high-cost decedents, perhaps some would regard the expenditures on the decedents as wasteful or unnecessary. However, such prospective distinctions are usually problematic, especially in cases that are likely to involve high costs. In short, even for those who may feel that in 1987 it was not worthwhile to spend $2.8 billion (or 0.6 percent of a national total of $500 billion) on high-cost Medicare decedents, there is no practicable way to put into effect a policy that would save such funds without also deliberately cutting off successful treatment for an equal number of likely survivors.

Predicting death very far in advance—12, 5, or 3 months in advance—with a high degree of certainty is largely beyond the present state of the art in medicine. As Scitovsky (1984) notes, the main exceptions are in the case of certain cancer patients, and it is no accident that hospices, generally less costly than hospitals, primarily serve such patients. Physicians' ability to predict mortality and to act on the basis of their predictions, however, is improving with respect to certain types of circumstances; for example, for a patient of advanced old age in an intensive care unit, with three organ systems failing, the odds of mortality are virtually 100 percent (Knaus et al., 1985). This kind of predictive information can be used confidently to support the withdrawal of medical treatment.

Medicine nonetheless remains more of a healing art than an exact science, and its focus is on human beings, not economic profit and loss. Consequently, some of the basic principles of applied economics, such as cost-benefit analysis and cost-effectiveness analysis, do not fit well in the health care arena (Avorn, 1984). For example, it might not make economic sense, prospectively and hypothetically, to treat a group of 100 very high cost patients when well-established probabilities indicate that only 20 of them will survive the year. However, for the physician, who is unable in such high-cost cases to be certain which persons will live, the undertaking cannot be viewed as a project doomed to failure simply because the net outcome will be 80 decedents and 20 survivors.

Medical Practice and the Geriatric Challenge

We are not aware of any extant proposals for rationing the health care of older persons that could—even putting aside ethical and moral issues—practicably be implemented as reforms in the practice of contemporary American medicine and constrain costs significantly. It is possible, of course, that cost-containment concerns may ultimately lead our governments, even our federal government, to follow the general precedent that is being set by Alameda County and the state of Oregon in their Medicaid programs and draw up official regulations denying Medicaid and/or Medicare reimbursement for specific medical interventions undertaken for persons beyond a certain old age.

Whether or not some form of official age-based rationing of medical care ever becomes palatable politically, the growing geriatric needs outlined earlier pose enormous economic and medical challenges. Are there other ways to approach those challenges than through explicitly age-discriminatory allocation patterns? We think so.

Responsible Medicine

First, society can reasonably expect the profession of medicine to be responsive to some specific issues. How can useful medical care that serves the values of the older patient be delivered in a way that is reasonable and sensitive to costs? To do this the medical profession and society must clarify mutually the obligations of physicians to patients and how those obligations are considered at the bedside, where clinical decision making occurs. These obligations should incorporate at least several elements.

Medical care must be efficacious if applied to a patient in a given circumstance. For a 70-year-old individual with end-stage Alzheimer's disease, pneumonia, and heart failure, the undertaking of cardiopulmonary resuscitation is essentially futile (Bedell et al., 1983). For an otherwise healthy 95-year-old who manifests a cardiac condition, a pacemaker might be a very useful intervention both to preserve longevity and maintain a high quality of life. Clinical research continues to clarify which persons are likely to benefit from specific interventions.

Medical care must be consonant with the patient's wishes. Western culture consistently affirms the right of the competent adult to refuse even life-sustaining treatment. Interventions must be made only with the patient's consent, if the patient is able to give consent.

Medical interventions must meet a test of reasonableness both to the individual and the physicians involved. It might be "reasonable" for a 90-year-old woman to decline to have a life-saving amputation or to refuse cardiopulmonary resuscitation, and for her physician to accept her wishes, on the basis of the patient's own personal values and her views regarding her remaining months or years. It would not be reasonable for a physician to accept the expressed wish of a 60-year-old woman to have a mastectomy because of her fear of developing breast cancer, or to accept a clinically depressed 20-year-old's refusal to undergo life-saving therapy.

The "Geriatric-Sensitive" Model of Medical Practice

The model of care most widely used in American medicine has a strong biomedical/disease orientation that emphasizes a sequential process: obtaining the patient's history; undertaking a physical examination; making a diagnosis; and recommending treatment. Although there are some recommended models of medical decision making that explicitly call for attention to the patient's values (e.g., Thomasma, 1978), for most practitioners such matters customarily remain secondary to the biomedical facts of the case.

The traditional model has been quite satisfactory in most circumstances, particularly when it can reasonably be assumed that the patient's objective is to be cured and that he or she is willing to have any treatment needed for survival. This approach continues to have utility for most persons with an acute, single-system illness such as a broken bone, acute appendicitis, pneumonia, or cardiac arrest (in a previously healthy person).

For aged persons with multiple interacting illnesses, however, this model is often unsatisfactory. As suggested earlier, many unfortunate instances of inappropriate, painful, and/or needlessly costly treatment of older persons result from a lack of adequate prior discussions among physicians, patients, and the patients' family members, as well as from poor prognostic information. The need for such discussions and information, and their documentation, is particularly important when "sentinel" changes in health status or care arrangements take place, such as the development of a serious progressive illness, the prospect of a major surgical intervention, or entrance to a nursing home. Even the passage of an advanced birthday, such as the eightieth, is often a good cause in itself for gathering information and undertaking value discussions.

A "geriatric-sensitive" model of care that includes doctor-patient-family discussions and prognostic information is essential for anticipating catastrophic changes in health status and making decisions that both are therapeutically optimal and avoid needless human agony and unnecessary costs. Through this painstaking process of gathering data and information, geriatricians, in their primary care and consultative roles, are already refining the traditional model of medical decision making to better serve the circumstances of older patients, and are teaching this model to medical students.

An important concept inherent in any geriatric model for clinical care is the recognition that there is a natural life span and that death eventually becomes inevitable as an outcome. With advancing age, the risk of death from nearly all particular causes increases, and the aggregate risk also increases exponentially (Manton, 1990). Even elimination of the top three causes of death at present (heart disease, cancer, and stroke) would only increase the relative importance of other causes of mortality. Death can only be postponed, not eliminated. In the context of the medical care provided to individuals, there is always some point at which cure, or even the prevention of death, is not possible.

The inevitability of death, of course, is the source of much of the discussion regarding the issues involved in finding a balance between the prolongation of life at all costs, and the preservation of the quality of life. These issues cannot be resolved categorically and *a priori*, without reference to the individual patient's specific values and definitions of "quality of life," as well as to the specific clinical realities of his or her circumstances.

Thus, the refinements of the geriatric-sensitive model call for a highly individualistic orientation, taking into account the unique characteristics of each patient within the context of a doctor-patient-family relationship. Using this undramatic approach, physicians can make recommendations and decisions that respect the values and the preferences of older patients (Jahnigen and Schrier, 1986) and make effective use of health care resources. The essential elements of the geriatric refinement of traditional medical decision making can be outlined as follows:

1. Value inventory. This initial phase is best undertaken well in advance of "sentinel changes," over time and within the primary care relationship. It is an attempt to ascertain the patient's value system. Information is gathered on such issues as whether or not the patient is religious, whether he or she is a "risk taker," and how he or she perceives his or her present quality of life and the course of life remaining. Family members can often contribute valuable information if the patient is unable to do so. Records are also made of existing formal plans or documents regarding the patient's wishes with respect to aggressive medical care and life-sustaining technologies.

2. *Determination of the patient's goals.* Patients come to medical care seeking a variety of outcomes. These are not always explicit. The physician and the patient both have an obligation to make sure that they are fully understood. Although some patients seek a cure, others seek an explanation of symptoms, reassurance, rehabilitation, palliation, or even sympathy from the physician (Wanzer et al., 1984; Wanzer et al., 1989). Often a combination of goals is involved. It is essential that the physician understand what patients seem to want for themselves before making medical recommendations.

3. *Medical and functional assessment.* In this step of the process, a history of the symptoms, the physical examination, the available laboratory data, and a functional assessment are incorporated into a differential diagnosis. Out of this, a primary diagnosis (or diagnoses) is made, and an attempt is made to determine the prognosis for the condition(s). Therapeutic options are considered within the context of the risk/benefit ratio for each specific patient and the patient's expressed values and objectives.

4. *Diagnosis or therapeutic recommendations.* The patient should have a full opportunity to consider the physician's recommendations and to express agreement or disagreement. Since family members often have an important investment in the implications of such recommendations, their active participation in this phase should be encouraged. As the physician's recommendations may differ from what is ultimately acceptable to the patient, compromise is often necessary. For instance, the physician might recommend radical, potentially curative surgery, while the patient will only accept conservative treatment that is less effective but eliminates a long postoperative period of extended hospitalization and recuperation. The physician might then respond by recommending a minor surgical procedure that would offer symptomatic relief, but not cure. Similarly, education by the physician regarding the implications of a specific recommendation may be important in resolving patient-family tensions regarding a proposed course of therapy. Family members may be helped, for example, to accept an older person's choice of conservative or palliative care, or a decision to remain at home alone, with risk of injury, rather than to enter a nursing home.

5. *Objective of care.* In this final step, an objective for care is developed, upon which the patient, family, and physician agree. The objective(s) of care is made clear, and measures of success are established. The objective may be complete cure of the condition (e.g., repair of a fracture), or it may be rehabilitation of function (e.g., following a stroke). It may be a diagnostic objective involving more detailed investigations that are necessary to determine fully the nature of the problem. It may be a prevention objective involving the use of immunization, physical strengthening, and/or improved nutrition to prevent future disability. Alternatively, the objective may be symptomatic relief of chronic disabling conditions such as incontinence, arthritis, or diabetes; or, when the patient has a terminal illness, palliation, using comfort measures to relieve distressing symptoms, can meet the objectives of preserving the patient's dignity and autonomy. In each case, the limitations and possibilities of medical care with respect to achieving the agreed-upon objectives should be made clear to the patient.

This highly individualized process can help make the use of medical technology more effective. Categorical age-based rationing, per se, has no place in this proccess. A focus on the individual provides an opportunity for the physician to inform patients and family members by providing realistic estimates of the utility and the success of treatments. At the point where the physician begins to withhold useful care *only* on the basis of cost, excluding efficacy, he or she is no longer the patient's advocate and has stepped outside the ethics of Western medicine (Angel, 1985; Levinsky, 1984).

The utility of this geriatric-sensitive model of medical practice could be substantially improved through additional research. Better information is needed on the medical efficacy of specific procedures when they are applied to subgroups of elderly persons. More reliable clinical predictors could be established for specific illnesses or combinations of illnesses. More effective methods of communication among physicians, patients, and families could be devised (Kohn, 1988); and public education regarding the usefulness or futility of medical interventions in various circumstances could help patients and their families to make more informed decisions (Fink et al., 1987).

Old Age, Rationing, and Justice

Even if the practice of American medicine becomes more refined to meet the geriatric challenges that lie ahead, it is doubtful that concerns about the financing of health care costs will subside in the United States. However, will these concerns remain so focused on older persons?

We hope not, because the practical implication of rationing on the basis of old age would be to deny many persons very effective therapies that can preserve life or restore function for a fairly long period of time. The value of such preservation and restoration is not confined to the older patients themselves but is usually also important to their family and friends, and others who treasure them.

Moreover, the contemporary tendency to frame issues of health care costs as matters of "justice between the young and the old" (see Daniels, 1988) is arbitrary, and diverts attention from other important health care issues. If we can put aside our preoccupation with Medicare and the age-categorical principle that it expresses, perhaps we will see that it is the capacity of patients to pay for charges—out-of-pocket or through third-party reimbursements—that has a great deal to do with the allocation of care.

What would happen if Medicare were totally eliminated? Wealthy, famous, and socially well-connected older persons would be able to obtain and/or pay for extensive and high-quality care out-of-pocket. Many more would be able to afford to pay premiums that would insure most of the costs of their care. Near-poor and poor older persons would be left in the same position as medically indigent persons of all ages.

In this light, we can more clearly see that explicit and formal age-based rationing, with its tacit judgments regarding the worthiness of human lives, would extend and deepen the traditional and strongly embedded American style of injustice: the distribution of health care resources (as well as, for example, educational resources) on the basis of social and economic class.

"Justice between rich and poor" may be a better metaphor than "justice between age groups" for the dilemmas of equity we might confront in the explicit rationing of health care. With the issue seen in this light, the specific policy options we might generate and consider would be rather different from those we are contemplating now, and would more likely reflect the true tradeoffs that do take place in the allocation of health care resources.

Political philosopher Michael Walzer (1983) has argued that throughout history, notions of justice have varied not only among cultures and political systems but also among distinct spheres of activity within any given culture or political system. Nothing requires Americans to devise or to accept separate spheres of justice within the health care arena, whether these would be defined on the basis of age, or whether they would separate the relatively wealthy from the relatively poor. We may prefer to delineate the health care arena as a distinct sphere of justice within which no such distinctions are made, and appropriate health care is provided to all.

The achievement of justice in providing health care, without rationing on the basis of demographic categories or economic class, is a political choice. The aggregate of resources that our nation devotes to health care is more than adequate to the task. Health economist Uwe Reinhardt explains the situation very clearly: "If the American public, and the politicians who represent it, really cared about the nation's indigent, they ought to be able to exploit the emerging surplus of health care resources to the advantage of the poor" (1986, p. 29). This challenge, in our view, is by far the most important to be addressed with respect to the future of American health care and the preservation and enhancement of the moral fabric of American society.

References

Aaron, H.J., and Schwartz, W.B. (1984). *The painful prescription: rationing hospital care.* Washington, D.C.: Brookings Institution.

Aaron, H.J., and Schwartz, W.B. (1990). Rationing health care: the choice before us. *Science, 247,* 418–422.

Abel-Smith, B. (1985). Who is the odd man out? the experience of Western Europe in containing the costs of health care. *Milbank Memorial Fund Quarterly/Health and Society, 63,* 1–17.

American Medical Association (1984). *Physician opinion on health care issues.* Chicago: Survey & Opinion Research.

Angel, M. (1985). Cost containment and the physician. *Journal of the American Medical Association, 254,* 1203–1207.

Areen, J. (1987). The legal status of consent obtained from families of adult patients to withhold or withdraw treatment. *Journal of the American Medical Association, 258,* 229–235.

Avorn, J. (1984). Benefit and cost analysis in geriatric care. *New England Journal of Medicine, 310,* 1294–1301.

Barber, J. (1989). Sick to death: caught between rising costs and more restraints, hospitals are cutting services. *Maclean's,* February 13, pp. 32–35.

Barondess, J., Kalb, P., Weil, W., Cassel, C., and Ginzberg, E. (1988). Clinical decision-making in catastrophic situations: the relevance of age. *Journal of the American Geriatrics Society, 36,* 919–937.

Bedell, S., Delbanco, T., Cook, E., and Epstein, F. (1983). Survival after cardiopulmonary resuscitation in the hospital. *New England Journal of Medicine, 309,* 569–576.

Besdine, R. (1980). Geriatric medicine. In C. Eisdorfer, ed., *Annual review of gerontology and geriatrics,* vol. 1, pp. 135–153. New York: Springer Publishing Co.

Blakeslee, S. (1989). Data suggest that implants may pose risk of later harm. *New York Times,* July 25, p. 17.

Blank, R.H. (1988). *Rationing medicine.* New York: Columbia University Press.

Brody, J.A. (1989). Toward quantifying the health of the elderly. *American Journal of Public Health, 79,* 685–686.

Burns, R., Graney, M., and Nichols, L. (1989). Predictors of in-hospital cardiopulmonary arrest outcome. *Archives of Internal Medicine, 149,* 1318–1321.

Callahan, D. (1987). *Setting limits: medical goals in an aging society.* New York: Simon & Schuster.

Callahan, D. (1990). *What kind of life: the limits of medical progress.* New York: Simon & Schuster.

Churchill, L.R. (1987). *Rationing health care in America: perceptions and principles of justice.* Notre Dame, Ind.: University of Notre Dame Press.

Committee on an Aging Society, Institute of Medicine, and National Research Council (1985). *Health in an older society.* Washington, D.C.: National Academy Press.

Daniels, N. (1988). *Am I my parents' keeper? an essay on justice between the young and the old.* New York: Oxford University Press.

Danis, M., Patrick, D., Southerland, L., and Green, M. (1988). Patient's and families' preferences for medical intensive care. *Journal of the American Medical Association, 260,* 797–802.

Edmunds, L.H., Stephenson, L., Edie, R., and Ratcliffe, M. (1988). Open-heart surgery in octogenarians. *New England Journal of Medicine, 319,* 131–136.

Enthoven, A. (1989). A "cost-unconscious" medical system. *New York Times,* July 13, p. 19.

Fink, A., Siu, A., Brook, R., Park, R., and Solomon, D. (1987). Assuring the quality of health care for older persons: an expert panel's priorities. *Journal of the American Medical Association, 258,* 1905–1908.

Freudenheim, M. (1989a). Calling for a bigger U.S. health role. *New York Times,* May 30, p. 29.

Freudenheim, M. (1989b). Debating Canadian health "model." *New York Times,* June 29, p. 27.

Freudenheim, M. (1989c). A health-care taboo is broken. *New York Times,* May 8, p. 23.

Fries, J.F. (1987). An introduction to the compression of morbidity. *Gerontologica Perspecta, 1,* 5–8.

Fries, J., and Crapo, L. (1981). *Vitality and aging.* San Francisco: W.H. Freeman.

Garland, S.B. (1989). Health care for all or an excuse for cutbacks? *Business Week,* June 26, p. 68.

Gillick, M. (1988). Limiting medical care: physicians' beliefs, physicians' behavior. *Journal of the American Geriatrics Society, 36,* 747–752.

Gordon, M., and Hurowitz, E. (1984). Cardiopulmonary resuscitation of the elderly. *Journal of the American Geriatrics Society, 32,* 930–934.

Gornick, M., Greenberg, J.N., Eggers, P.W., and Dobson, A. (1985). Twenty years of Medicare and Medicaid: covered populations, use of benefits, and program expenditures. *Health Care Financing Review, annual suppl.,* p. 22.

Grimes, D.S. (1987). Rationing health care. *Lancet, 1*(8533), 615–616.

Gross, J. (1989). What medical care the poor can have: lists are drawn up. *New York Times,* March 27, p. 1.

Health Care Financing Administration (1987). National health expenditures, 1986–2000. *Health Care Financing Review, 8*(4), 1–36.

Hiatt, H.H. (1987). *America's health in the balance: choice or change?* New York: Harper & Row.

Hing, E. (1987). *Use of nursing homes by the elderly: preliminary data from the 1985 National Nursing Home Survey.* Advance Data no. 135. Hyattsville, Md.: National Center for Health Statistics, May 14.

Hosking N., Warner, M., Lobdell, C., Offord, K., and Melton, J., III (1989). Outcomes of surgery in patients 90 years of age and older. *Journal of the American Medical Association, 261,* 1909–1915.

Iglehart, J.K. (1986). Canada's health care system. *New England Journal of Medicine, 313,* 202–208, 778–784, and 1623–1628.

Jahnigen, D., and Schrier, R. (1986). The doctor-patient relationship in geriatric care. In D. Jahnigen and R. Schrier, eds., *Ethical issues in the care of the elderly,* pp. 457–464. Philadelphia: W.B. Saunders.

Katz, S., Branch, L.G., Branson, M.H., Papsidero, J.A., Beck, J.C., and Greer, D.S. (1983). Active life expectancy. *New England Journal of Medicine, 309,* 1218–1224.

Kinzer, D.M. (1983). Massachusetts and California—two kinds of hospital cost control. *New England Journal of Medicine, 308,* 838–841.

Kleiman, D. (1985). Death and the court. *New York Times,* January 19, p. 9.

Knaus, W., Draper, E., Wagner, D., and Zimmerman, J. (1985). Prognosis in acute organ system failure. *Annals of Surgery, 302,* 685–693.

Koenig, R. (1986). As liver transplants grow more common, ethical issues multiply: by operating on the elderly, Thomas Starzl steps up patient selection debate. *Wall Street Journal,* October 14, p. 1.

Kohn, M., and Meno, G. (1988). Life prolongation: views of elderly outpatients and health care professionals. *Journal of the American Geriatrics Society, 36,* 840–844.

Labouvie-Vief, G. (1985). Intelligence and cognition. In J. Birren and W. Schaie, eds., *Handbook of the psychology of aging,* pp. 500–530. New York: Van Nostrand Reinhold.

Lamm, R.D. (1987). A debate: Medicare in 2020. In *Medicare reform and the Baby Boom generation,* edited proceedings of the second annual conference of Americans for Generational Equity, April 30–May 1, 1987, pp. 77–88. Washington, D.C.: Americans for Generational Equity.

Lamm, R.D. (1989). Columbus and Copernicus: new wine in old wineskins. *Mount Sinai Journal of Medicine, 56*(1), 1–10.

La Puma, J., Silverstein, M., Stocking, C., Roland, D., and Siegler, M. (1988). Life-sustaining treatment: a prospective study of patients with DNR orders in a teaching hospital. *Archives of Internal Medicine, 148,* 2193–2198.

Latta, V.B., and Helbing, C. (1988). Medicare: short-stay hospital services, by leading diagnosis-related groups, 1983–1985. *Health Care Financing Review, 10*(2), 79–107.

Lerner, H.M. (1990). Don't look to Canada's health system. *New York Times,* February 3, p. 17.

Letsch, S.W., Levit, K.R., and Waldo, D.R. (1988). National health expenditures, 1987. *Health Care Financing Review, 10*(2), 109–122.

Levinsky, N. (1984). The doctor's master. *New England Journal of Medicine*, *311*, 1573–1575.

Lo, B., and Jonsen, A. (1980). Clinical decisions to limit treatment. *Annals of Internal Medicine*, *93*, 764–768.

Loop, F., Lytle, B., Cosgrove, D., Goormastic, H., Taylor, P., Golding, L., Stewart, R., and Gill, C. (1988). Coronary artery bypass graft surgery in the elderly. *Cleveland Clinic Journal of Medicine*, *55*, 23–24.

Lubitz, J., and Prihoda, R. (1984). The use and costs of Medicare services in the last two years of life. *Health Care Financing Review*, *5*(3), 117–131.

Manton, K.G. (1990). Mortality and morbidity. In R.H. Binstock and L.K. George, eds., *Handbook of aging and the social sciences* (3rd ed.), pp. 64–90. San Diego: Academic Press.

Mechanic, D. (1985a). Cost containment and the quality of medical care: rationing strategies in an era of constrained resources. *Milbank Memorial Fund Quarterly/Health and Society*, *63*, 453–475.

Mechanic, D. (1985b). Public perceptions of medicine. *New England Journal of Medicine*, *321*, 181–183.

Miles, S., and Ryder, M. (1985). Limited-treatment policies in long-term care facilities. *Journal of the American Geriatrics Society*, *33*, 707.

National Center for Health Statistics (1987a). *Current estimates from the National Health Interview Survey, United States, 1986.* Series 10, no. 164. Hyattsville, Md.: U.S. Department of Health and Human Services.

National Center for Health Statistics (1987b). *Health United States, 1986.* Pub. no. (PHS) 87-1232. Hyattsville, Md.: U.S. Department of Health and Human Services.

National Center for Health Statistics (1987c). Utilization of short-stay hospitals, United States, 1985, annual summary. *Vital and Health Statistics*, Series 13, no. 91. Hyattsville, Md.: U.S. Department of Health and Human Services, May.

Nye, J.S., Jr. (1990). The misleading metaphor of decline. *Atlantic*, *265*(3), 86–94.

Okrent, D. (1987). You and the doctor: striving for a better relationship. *New York Times*, March 29, p. 20.

Pearlman, R., Inui, T., and Carter, W. (1982). Variability in physician bioethical decision-making. *Annals of Internal Medicine*, *97*, 420–425.

Reinhardt, U.E. (1986). Letter of June 9, 1986, to Arnold S. Relman. *Health Affairs*, *5*(2), 28–31.

Robinson, D. (1989). Who should receive medical aid? *Parade*, May 28, p. 4.

Roos, N.P., Montgomery, P., and Roos, L.L. (1987). Health care utilization in the years prior to death. *Milbank Memorial Fund Quarterly/Health and Society*, *65*, 231–254.

Rowe, J. (1977). Clinical research on aging: strategies and new directions. *New England Journal of Medicine*, *292*, 1332–1336.

Rowe, J., Andres, R., Tobin, J., Norris, A., and Shock, N. (1976). The effects of age on creatinine clearance in man. *Journal of Gerontology*, *31*, 155–163.

Rowe, J., and Binstock, R. (1987). Aging reconsidered: emerging research and policy issues. In E. Ginzberg, ed., *Medicine and society: clinical decisions and societal values*, pp. 96–113. Boulder, Colo.: Westview Press.

Ruark, J., Raffin, T., and the Stanford University Medical Center Committee on Ethics (1988). Initiating and withdrawing life support: principles and practice in adult medicine. *New England Journal of Medicine, 318,* 25–30.

Rudman, D., Feller, A.G., Nagraj, H.S., Gergans, G.A., Lalitha, P.Y., Goldberg, A.F., Schlenker, R.A., Cohn, L., Rudman, I.W., and Mattson, D.E. (1990). Effects of human growth hormone in men over 60 years old. *New England Journal of Medicine, 323,* 1–6.

Sage, W., Hurst, C., Silverman, J., and Bortz, W., II (1987). Intensive care for the elderly: outcomes of elective and non-elective admissions. *Journal of the American Geriatrics Society, 35,* 312–318.

Schneider, E.L., and Guralnik, J.M. (1987). The compression of morbidity: a dream which may come true, someday! *Gerontologica Perspecta, 1,* 8–14.

Schneider, E.L., and Guralnik, J.M. (1990). The aging of America: impact on health care costs. *Journal of the American Medical Association, 263,* 2335–2340.

Schulte, J. (1983). Terminal patients deplete Medicare, Greenspan says. *Dallas Morning News,* April 26, p. 1.

Schwartz, D., and Reilly, P. (1986). The choice not to be resuscitated. *Journal of the American Geriatrics Society, 34,* 807–811.

Schwartz, W.B., and Aaron, H.J. (1985). Health care costs: the social tradeoffs. *Issues in Science and Technology, 1*(2), 39–46.

Scitovsky, A.A. (1984). "The high cost of dying": what do the data show? *Milbank Memorial Fund Quarterly/Health and Society, 62,* 591–608.

Scitovsky, A.A. (1988). Medical care in the last twelve months of life: the relation between age, functional status, and medical care expenditures. *Milbank Memorial Fund Quarterly/Health and Society, 66,* 640–660.

Shock, N.W., Greulich, R., Andres, R., Arenberg, D., Costa, P., Jr., Lakatta, E., and Tobin, J. (1984). *Normal human aging: the Baltimore longitudinal study of aging.* Washington, D.C.: U.S. Government Printing Office.

Smith, T. (1989). BMA rejects NHS review but . . . doctors must develop a coherent alternative. *British Medical Journal, 298,* 1405–1406.

Starr, P. (1982). *The social transformation of American medicine.* New York: Basic Books.

Taeuber, C. (1990). Diversity: the dramatic reality. In S. Bass, E. Kutza, and F. Torres-Gil, eds., *Diversity in aging: the issues facing the White House Conference on Aging and beyond*, pp. 1–45. Glenview, Ill.: Scott, Foresman & Co.

Thomasma, D. (1978). Training in medical ethics: an ethical workship. *Forum on Medicine, 1*(December), 33–36.

Thurow, L.C. (1985). Medicine versus economics. *New England Journal of Medicine, 313,* 611–614.

Tresch, D., Thakur, R., Hoffman, R., Olson, D., and Brooks, H. (1989). Should the elderly be resuscitated following out-of-hospital cardiac arrest? *American Journal of Medicine, 86,* 145–150.

U.S. Congress, Office of Technology Assessment (1987). *Life-sustaining technologies and the elderly.* Washington, D.C.: U.S. Government Printing Office.

U.S. House of Representatives, Select Committee on Aging (1989). *Health care costs for America's elderly, 1977–88.* Washington, D.C.: U.S. Government Printing Office.

U.S. Senate, Special Committee on Aging (1989). *Aging America: trends and projections.* Washington, D.C.: U.S. Government Printing Office.

Waldo, D., Levit, K., and Lazenby, H. (1986). National health expenditures, 1985. *Health Care Financing Review, 8*(1), 1–21.

Walker, M.A. (1989). From Canada: a different viewpoint. *Health Marketing Quarterly,* 1st qtr., pp. 11–13.

Walzer, M. (1983). *Spheres of justice.* New York: Basic Books.

Wanzer, S., Adelstein, S., Crandford, R., Federman, D., Hook, E., Moertel, C., Safar, P., Stone, A., Taussig, H., and van Eys, J. (1984). The physician's responsibility towards hopelessly ill patients. *New England Journal of Medicine, 310,* 955–959.

Wanzer, S., Federman, D., Adelstein, J., Cassel, C., Cassem, E., Cranford, R., Hook, E., Lo, B., Mortel, C., Safar, P., Stone, A., and van Eys, J. (1989). The physician's responsibility toward hopelessly ill patients: a second look. *New England Journal of Medicine, 320,* 844–849.

Watts, N.B., Harris, S.T., Genant, H.K., Wasnich, R.D., Miller, P.D., Jackson, R.D., Licata, A.A., Ross, P., Woodson, G.D., III, Yannover, M.J., Mysiw, W.J., Kohse, L., Rao, M.B., Steiger, P., Richmond, B., and Chesnut, C.H., III (1990). Intermittent cyclical etidronate treatment of postmenopausal osteoporosis. *New England Journal of Medicine, 323,* 73–79.

Whitney, C.R. (1989). Thatcher's new health plan: an outcry rises on all sides. *New York Times,* June 26, p. 1.

Youngner, S., Lewandowski, W., McClish, D., Juknialis, B., Coulton, C., and Bartlett, E. (1985). Do not resuscitate orders: incidence and implications in a medical intensive care unit. *Journal of the American Medical Association, 253,* 54–57.

3

Advanced Medical Technology and Elderly People

ROGER W. EVANS, Ph.D.

Despite abundant evidence that elderly persons are highly diverse physiologically, psychologically, and socially (Birren, 1986), chronological old age is a well-established focal point for discussions in the United States regarding the allocation of health care resources. For example, while the U.S. Congress, Office of Technology Assessment (OTA) recognizes that the elderly population is heterogeneous, it nonetheless legitimizes the usage of age 65 as an official marker:

> Sixty-five, or any chronological age, is a poor indicator of biological function, physiological reserve, cognitive ability, or health care needs. The use of 65 is justified, however, by its prominence in available health and demographic statistics and its relevance to eligibility criteria in current Federal and State health care programs, especially Medicare. (1987; p. 5)

Older Patients and the Use of Advanced Medical Technology

Defining who is considered "elderly" in relation to the use of advanced medical technology can be difficult. The application of such technology is a gradual process. Chronological age is often a consideration because of the ease with which it is determined, even though—according to many people—an individual's health status and probability of benefit are the real issues.

The correlation between chronological age and health status is often weak. As this is recognized, the chronological age limits placed on the use of new technology may be adjusted accordingly. For example, in

44

1967 only 7 percent of patients in the United States receiving kidney dialysis—a process for cleansing the blood of waste products—were aged 55 and over. By 1978, this percentage had increased to 46 percent, and by 1986, nearly 58 percent of all dialysis patients in this country were aged 55 and over (Evans et al., 1981; Health Care Financing Administration, 1989). In 1967 few people would have predicted that within two decades the majority of dialysis patients in the United States would be aged 55 and older. Even fewer would have believed that by 1986 10 percent of U.S. dialysis patients would be aged 75 and over. The experience with open heart surgery has been very similar to that with kidney dialysis. In 1965 few analysts would have predicted correctly that octogenarians would be subjected to complex open heart surgery including coronary artery bypass grafting, aortic valve replacement, and mitral valve replacement (Edmunds et al., 1988).

Clearly, the definition of *elderly* changes on the basis of the experience to date with a given technology. It is this very phenomenon that must be carefully monitored. The combined experience with the aforementioned technologies clearly indicates that some effort should be made to track the use of advanced medical technologies that have even a remote possibility of benefiting persons over the age of 60, so that they can be applied appropriately. Moreover, as criteria for the selection of patients are relaxed, even considerations related to the patient's health may become less influential when the application of certain technologies is contemplated. Kidney, heart, and liver transplantation are noteworthy examples of procedures for which the criteria have undergone such changes. Although these procedures are now considered established therapies for persons younger than 55 years of age, they are being used increasingly to treat patients over the age of 60. Subject to the availability of donor organs, it may well be that within the next decade a growing number of persons 60 years of age or older, regardless of health status, will benefit from organ transplantation.

Unfortunately, the use of advanced medical technologies may increasingly become complicated by concerns related to cost-effectiveness. It is widely believed that health care expenditures are out of control and that advanced technology has contributed greatly to rising expenditures. In this context, elderly patients may well be handicapped in gaining access to expensive medical technologies such as kidney dialysis and organ transplantation, since the benefits they derive may be of shorter duration than the benefits derived by younger patients (Avorn, 1984). The dilemma is obvious, yet the solution is unclear.

In some nations, various older ages are already widely used, unofficially, as an indication to deny health care that requires advanced technology. In the British National Health Service, for instance, general practitioners simply do not refer patients who have end-stage kidney diseases to kidney specialists for dialysis treatment if the patients are aged 55 or older (Aaron and Schwartz, 1984; Schwartz and Aaron, 1984).

In the United States, the application of such an age limit would reduce the size of the dialysis patient population by over 50 percent. Limiting patients' access to health care clearly has the potential to both reduce and constrain total health care expenditures. The real issue is not the effect of such limitations but rather, their palatability. It is unclear whether the sociopolitical environment of the United States would be receptive to instituting broad-based age discrimination in the interest of reducing national health care expenditures. The topic is up for discussion, however.

As medical technology has increased in both sophistication and cost, it has become commonplace for health care analysts and biomedical ethicists to raise questions regarding what constitutes an appropriate level of care for the elderly. They often argue, for example, that elderly people do not benefit maximally from procedures such as organ transplantation, coronary artery bypass grafts, kidney dialysis, cancer treatment, and other such advanced procedures (Callahan, 1988; Callahan, 1989; Colen, 1986; Daniels, 1987; Schneider, 1989). Many such analysts also contend that the quality of life of elderly persons is severely compromised, and that when assessed in terms of quality-adjusted life years, the elderly gain little from expensive medical technologies. Thus, it is argued that the use of these technologies in the treatment of elderly patients is unjustifiable from the perspective of benefit to the patient as well as cost.

This chapter specifically looks at the use of technologically advanced treatments for older patients and traces the evolution of three such treatments—kidney dialysis, kidney transplantation, and heart transplantation—in patients of all age groups. It examines the outcomes of these treatments for older patients and compares them with the outcomes for younger patients. The critical "gatekeeper" role played by the Medicare program in the development, the application, and the diffusion of such new technologies in our health care system is described briefly, and our limited knowledge of the overall costs of the widespread use of new technologies is outlined.

Older Patients and the Benefits of Advanced Technology: An Examination of Three Procedures

What, in fact, is the history of the use of advanced medical technologies in the treatment of older persons? Do older patients benefit from the use of these technologies? If so, how do they fare by comparison with younger patients?

Some older persons unquestionably benefit from the application of very advanced medical technologies, such as kidney dialysis, kidney transplantation, and heart transplantation. There are no medical grounds for excluding elderly persons, categorically, as candidates for these treatments. If an older person's general health status is acceptable, he or she may well benefit from sophisticated medical and surgical procedures. As is the case with the broader range of medical interventions discussed in chapter 2, old age per se is not an important predictor of the success of treatment.

A good picture of how advanced technologies are applied for older patients, and how the patients benefit, can be gleaned from a detailed review of experiences with specific technologies. (However, it should be kept in mind that the definition of the "elderly" patient changes with the use of technology.) It is of particular interest to examine three technologies that are in different stages of development and utilization: kidney dialysis, kidney transplantation, and heart transplantation. Kidney dialysis is an established therapy for persons of all ages with kidney failure. Kidney transplantation is also an established therapy, although patient selection is in a transitional period. Some of the patients receiving transplants now are older and/or sicker than would have been acceptable five years ago. Within about five years, the average age of kidney transplant recipients has increased by 10 years. Finally, patients over the age of 50 have only recently begun to benefit from heart transplantation, the last of the three technologies examined here. Based upon the present age-utilization relationship, and without regard to health status, an elderly dialysis patient is defined as being 65 years of age or older, an elderly kidney transplant recipient is defined as being 60 years of age or over, and an elderly heart transplant recipient is defined as being 55 years of age or older.

Kidney Dialysis

Nearly one hundred thousand Americans are now receiving some form of kidney dialysis. When dialysis first became available as a standard therapy for life-threatening "kidney failure," or end-stage renal disease (ESRD), many older persons who could conceivably have benefited were excluded from consideration for treatment because of their advanced age (Evans et al., 1981). The main objective was to treat those persons who were the primary breadwinners within stable family households. Hence, persons over the age of 55 were often excluded from treatment (Evans et al., 1981; U.S. Congress, Office of Technology Assessment, 1987). The criteria used to select patients were essentially based on "social worth," and as a result, women, minorities, and persons with little education were often denied dialysis (Evans et al., 1989).

Today, however, due to the extension of Medicare benefits in 1973 to all persons with ESRD, virtually every American in need of treatment receives therapy regardless of age, social status, or ability to pay. This has had a marked impact on the sociodemographic characteristics of the kidney dialysis patient population, as apparent in Table 3.1, which

Table 3.1
Social and Demographic Characteristics of the Kidney Dialysis Patient Population, 1967 and 1978

Characteristic	Year	
	1967	*1978*
Sex		
Male	75	49.2
Female	25	50.8
Race		
White	91	63.7
Black	7	34.9
Other	2	1.4
Education		
Junior high school or less	10	28.7
Some high school	17	17.2
High school graduate	27	28.4
Some college	20	18.2
College graduate	12	5.7
Postgraduate school	13	1.8
Unknown	1	0.0
Age (years)		
<25	8	3.4
25–34	24	10.0
35–44	32	14.6
45–54	27	25.8
≥55	7	45.7
Unknown	2	0.5
Marital status		
Single	16	13.0
Married	79	61.8
Other	5	25.2

Source: Evans et al., 1981, p. 188. Copyright 1981, American Medical Association.

compares the patient population in 1967 with that in 1978. Whereas in 1967 only 7 percent of dialysis patients were aged 55 or over, today persons aged 65 and over are the fastest-growing age group in the dialysis population, increasing at an average annual rate of over 15 percent in recent years. In 1974, patients 65 and over who were eligible for Medicare ESRD benefits made up less than 5 percent of the average annual enrollment. By 1985, patients in this older age group accounted for more than 31 percent of Medicare's ESRD enrollees (Table 3.2) and 36 percent of new enrollees during the year (Health Care Financing Administration, 1988). Moreover, the age-group distribution of new patients enrolled into the ESRD program in 1985 indicates that the percentage of patients of advanced old age is becoming greater than it was in the past; whereas persons aged 75 and older were 9.4 percent of all ESRD enrollees in 1985 (Table 3.2), they were 11.9 percent of newly enrolled patients in that year (Table 3.3).

The expenditures of the ESRD program have escalated sharply since the program's inception. In 1974, they totaled $229 million. By 1980 they had more than quintupled to $1.3 billion, and they now approach $3 billion annually. This steep rise in program expenditures appears to be attributable to the increased number of beneficiaries rather than to sharp increases in per-patient treatment costs. Although the average annual Medicare reimbursement per enrollee (for dialysis patients and transplantation patients combined) increased from $14,300 in 1974 to $20,229 in 1980, by 1987 it had dropped slightly, to $20,213 (Evans et al., 1989). Thus, while program expenditures have increased markedly over the years, the reimbursement per enrollee has remained essentially unchanged since 1980. Nonetheless, the magnitude of the overall cost increases in the ESRD program has engendered alarm among

Table 3.2
Percentage of Enrollees, in Older Age Groups, in Medicare End-Stage Renal Disease Program, 1980–1985

Year	Percentage of Enrollees Aged 65 Years and Over	Percentage of Enrollees Aged 65–74 Years	Percentage of Enrollees Aged 75 Years and Over
1980	23.5	18.2	5.3
1981	24.4	18.6	5.8
1982	25.9	19.4	6.5
1983	28.5	20.7	7.8
1984	30.0	21.4	8.6
1985	31.4	22.0	9.4

Source: Health Care Financing Administration, 1988, p. 8.

Table 3.3
Percentage of New Enrollees, in Older Age Groups, in Medicare End-Stage Renal Disease Program, 1980–1985

Year	Percentage of Enrollees Aged 65 Years and Over	Percentage of Enrollees Aged 65–74 Years	Percentage of Enrollees Aged 75 Years and Over
1980	27.7	20.4	7.3
1981	27.7	20.4	7.3
1982	29.3	21.0	8.3
1983	35.0	23.9	11.1
1984	34.3	23.1	11.2
1985	35.9	24.0	11.9

Source: Health Care Financing Administration, 1988, p. 3.

Table 3.4
Percentage Distribution of Dialysis Patients, by Age and Length of Survival, 1982–1985

| Age (years) | Length of Survival | | |
	1 Year	2 Years	3 Years
<15	95.2	91.3	89.0
15–24	95.1	90.2	86.7
25–34	91.5	82.4	74.1
35–44	89.7	79.2	69.7
45–54	86.5	73.3	62.1
55–64	79.3	63.4	50.5
65–74	67.3	48.6	35.2
≥75	57.7	36.8	23.0
All ages	78.2	65.2	50.1

Source: Health Care Financing Administration, 1988, p. 28.

health care analysts. Some have suggested that the elderly be excluded from treatment because they do not benefit from treatment as much as younger persons do (Moskop, 1987).

It is true that the average survival rates of elderly patients receiving dialysis are lower than those of younger patients. As Table 3.4 shows for the years 1982 through 1985, the one-, two-, and three-year average survival rates for older patients are not as favorable as those for patients in younger categories. However, the rates are affected by factors other than age, such as the primary cause of kidney failure and whether or not the patient has additional illnesses at the time dialysis therapy is initiated. For example, ESRD patients of all ages for whom diabetes was the cause of renal failure had a one-year survival rate in 1985 of only 74.3 percent. This was more than 10 percent lower than the rate for ESRD patients generally (Health Care Financing Administration, 1988).

Thus, regardless of age, poor health adversely effects the outcome of dialysis. While age and poor health may be correlated, the relationship is not necessarily causal. Consequently, age is little more than a proxy indicator of health status and an imprecise predictor of benefit. The interaction of age and health status should be given greater weight than age alone.

Most analysts agree, however, that survival is not the only treatment benefit that should be assessed. For instance, in the National Kidney Dialysis and Kidney Transplantation Study, quality-of-life data were obtained for 859 ESRD dialysis patients (Evans et al., 1985; Evans et al., 1987). Although the data are not representative of the entire population of dialysis and transplant patients in the United States, they do represent a reasonably good age distribution of patients, thus providing some insights not available from other sources: 13 percent of the patients were aged 65 or older; of these, more than half were between the ages of 65 and 69, half as many again were aged 70 to 74, and the rest were aged 75 or older. Accordingly, a special report analyzing age-group comparisons in these data was commissioned by an OTA panel on life-sustaining technologies and the elderly (U.S. Congress, Office of Technology Assessment, 1987).

This analysis for OTA showed that older dialysis patients were faring relatively well in terms of quality-of-life measures. In comparison with younger ESRD patients, those aged 65 and over were shown by tests using the semantic differential approach to measurement to have higher self-reported well-being, more positive feelings, fewer negative feelings, and the view that life was more "easy" than "hard." They also were more satisfied with life in general and with their marriages, family lives, savings and investments, and standards of living, in particular.

On some other measures of the quality of life, however, these older persons did not fare as well. These results were consistent with overall comparisons between the older and younger segments of the U.S. population, and with the fact that elderly dialysis patients are—by definition—not in good health. The older patients expectably reported greater functional impairment than did the younger patients, markedly less ability to work, and a much lower current employment rate. Differences between the older and the younger patients with respect to self-reported capacity for the activities of daily living were, for the most part, negligible. However, not surprisingly, the older dialysis patients assessed their own health as poorer than that of others their age.

Despite this analysis, which suggests that the quality of life among older dialysis patients is reasonably good, there is also some evidence that they choose to withdraw from treatment at an unusually high rate. In one study, voluntary treatment withdrawal was the cause of death in 40 percent of patients aged 65 and older, compared with only 22 percent for all ages (Neu and Kjellstrand, 1986). In another study, conducted at the Regional Kidney Disease Center in Minnesota from 1966 to 1983, it was found that dialysis was voluntarily discontinued by 1 patient of every 11 in general, but by 1 of every 6 over age 60 (Lowance, 1988). Thus, the results of these studies suggest that although most older dialysis patients report a quality of life comparable to that of younger patients, some do not, in fact, necessarily find their life sufficiently satisfying to continue treatment and thereby avoid death.

Overall, then, the evidence suggests that selected elderly patients benefit from dialysis. However, the degree to which they are found to benefit depends on the relative weight given to different types of benefits. Clearly, the average survival rate is somewhat less for older ESRD patients than for younger ones. At the same time, in the aggregate, older patients seem to appreciate the quality of their remaining lives somewhat more than do younger patients, within the broader contexts of their general health and societal status. However, older patients seem more ready than younger ones to voluntarily withdraw from ongoing treatment with kidney dialysis.

Eventually it will be necessary to come to terms with what society can justifiably expect of dialysis patients. For many patients, particularly those who are retired or disabled, productivity is an inappropriate indicator of social worth. Similarly, while functional ability is a relevant endpoint and a geriatric concern, it is evident that dialysis patients are not necessarily more debilitated than persons of an equivalent age in the general population. Thus, their subjective experience with life may be the only acceptable indicator of benefit. If, however, society insists that independence and productivity are to be weighted more heavily, then the basis of such judgments must be recognized for what it is—the ascription of the value of an individual to society. On virtually all indicators of social worth, elderly persons, regardless of their health status, tend to be judged less worthy than younger persons.

Kidney Transplantation

Of the various treatments available for ESRD, kidney transplantation is considered the most effective (Evans et al., 1985; Evans et al., 1987). The clinical benefits, in terms of restored kidney function, are superior to those of any form of dialysis; and the quality of life experienced by patients is considerably better. Kidney transplant recipients whose new organs function satisfactorily also incur far lower treatment expenses than do dialysis patients (Evans et al., 1987; Evans et al., 1989).

For example, in a recently completed study the average cost of a kidney transplant was found to be $41,045. Average annual follow-up costs, including outpatient medications, range between $6,000 and $11,000 per patient. Alternatively, the average annual per-patient treatment cost for dialysis is at least $25,000 (Evans et al., 1989). Thus, over the expected life course of an ESRD patient, kidney transplantation—if successful—is the treatment modality that is most cost-effective per year of life saved.

Traditionally, kidney transplantation was virtually ruled out for patients of advanced age. For a transplantation to be successful, drug therapy to suppress the natural tendency of the body's immune system to reject foreign tissue (such as transplanted organs) was required; this therapy adversely affected mortality and morbidity rates among patients of all ages. Because the immune systems of patients at advanced ages generally tend to be weaker than those of younger persons, it was argued that older persons would have an especially difficult time withstanding the immunosuppressive therapy essential for transplantation. Therefore, it was projected that elderly patients would have greater morbidity and a higher mortality rate than did younger transplant recipients (Kock et al., 1980; Maver et al., 1989; Offner et al., 1989; Ost et al., 1980; Wedel et al., 1980).

This traditional rationale, however, has been countered by the recent experience of many transplant teams, particularly since the introduction in 1980 of cyclosporine, a highly effective drug for suppressing the immune system, which carries a reduced risk of adverse long-term side effects. Precisely because the immune system tends to be weaker in older patients, many elderly transplant recipients require smaller dosages of immunosuppressive agents in order to achieve the level of immune response that will minimize the likelihood of rejection of the transplanted organ. This is true for both kidney and heart transplantation.

Consequently, it is not surprising that numerous published reports have appeared in the literature arguing that advanced age should no longer be considered an absolute criterion for ruling out transplantation (Brynger et al., 1986; Cardella et al., 1989; Fehrman et al., 1989; Fryd et al., 1987; Howard et al., 1989; Ito et al., 1986; Lauffer et al., 1988; Murie et al., 1989; Pirsch et al., 1989; Shah et al., 1988). Thus, while in 1985 only 12 percent of all patients receiving transplants from cadaver organs were aged 55 or over (Table 3.5), it is possible, if there is an increase in the supply of donor organs available from cadavers,

Table 3.5
Medicare Beneficiaries Receiving Kidney Transplants, by Age of Patient and Type of Donor, 1985

Age of Patient (years)	Cadaver Donor		Living, Related Donor	
	Number	Percentage	Number	Percentage
0–14	187	4	168	10
15–24	590	12	327	20
25–34	1182	23	537	32
35–44	1435	28	348	21
45–54	1102	22	208	13
55–64	534	11	63	4
65–74	50	1	3	0
≥75	4	0	0	0
Average age	38.8		31.5	

Source: Eggers, 1988, p. 225. Reprinted by permission of the *New England Journal of Medicine*.

that this percentage could be augmented considerably in the future. Unfortunately, the supply of donor kidneys has remained stable over the past four years. Efforts to increase the supply have had virtually little impact. This has prompted an increased interest in relaxing the clinical contraindications for organ donation, even to the point of raising the maximum age of kidney donation to 70 years (Evans, 1990).

In effect, now that considerable experience has been accumulated in using cyclosporine as an immunosuppressive drug, kidney transplantation for older patients has come to be viewed as a viable and effective treatment. In the "precyclosporine era," the one-year patient survival rate and the organ survival rate for transplant recipients aged 60 and over averaged between 57 and 62 percent (Kock et al., 1980; Ost et al., 1980; Pirsch et al., 1989; Wedel et al., 1980). Many of these patients died of cardiac disease or infection. In general, transplant teams were discouraged by these results and tended to exclude elderly persons from consideration as candidates for transplantation. Shortly after the introduction of cyclosporine, in the years 1982 through 1985, the average one-year survival rate for persons aged 65 to 74 years had improved to 77.5 percent (Health Care Financing Administration, 1988). This improvement was sufficient to make the survival rates for older transplant patients substantially better than the survival rates of dialysis patients in the same age group (compare Tables 3.4 and 3.6).

A group at the University of Wisconsin has recently reported even better results from their kidney transplantation experience with patients

Table 3.6
Percentage Distribution of Patients after Kidney Transplant from Cadaver Donor, by Age and Length of Survival, 1982–1985

Age (years)	Length of Survival		
	1 Year	2 Years	3 Years
<15	95.1	92.9	89.1
15–24	95.2	92.4	89.0
25–34	93.0	89.2	84.7
35–44	90.7	85.5	80.3
45–54	87.2	81.6	76.7
55–64	83.4	75.9	68.0
65–74	77.5[a]	73.3[a]	67.9[a]
≥75	—[b]	—[b]	—[b]
All patients	90.6	85.9	81.1

Source: Health Care Financing Administration, 1988, p. 29.
[a] Based on 120 cases.
[b] Only 8 transplants performed.

aged between 60 and 73—averaging 62.8 years of age—undertaken in the cyclosporine era (Pirsch et al., 1989). They performed 36 transplants on such patients, using the most advanced techniques of immunosuppressive therapy. Most of the patients (88 percent) were on dialysis prior to transplantation, and 29 percent had atherosclerotic cardiovascular disease, or "hardening of the arteries." The Wisconsin team reported that the average three-year survival rate for their patients was 91 percent; the three-year survival rate for transplanted kidneys was 74 percent. Surgical complications were infrequent. Postoperatively, threatened "rejections" of the transplants were less frequent in these older patients than in younger ones, but were more likely to lead to loss of the transplanted organs. Medical complications, especially infection, were common after transplantation but were easily managed.

Based on their results, the Wisconsin group concluded that "renal transplantation with cyclosporine is a safe and effective therapeutic modality that is no longer contraindicated in elderly patients" (Pirsch et al., 1989, p. 259). In explaining this conclusion, they pointed out that age continues to be an important predictor of survival in patients who have begun dialysis, with a fourfold increase in the risk of mortality as the age at which dialysis is started increases from 25 to 65 years (see Mailloux et al., 1988).

Clearly, as this report and many others have shown, some elderly patients can benefit from kidney transplantation (Canadian Transplant Study Group, 1985; Cardella et al., 1989; Gordon et al., 1987; Ito et al., 1986; Murie et al., 1989). Some observers (e.g., Castro, 1986) still suggest that patients over 70 may have a poor prognosis for survival. Others are more optimistic, emphasizing that in considering older patients for transplants "adequate selection principles must be followed, basically those aimed at the biologic age, not the chronologic age, of the patient" (Brynger et al., 1986, p. 13).

Unfortunately, the number of elderly patients who can benefit from kidney transplantation may be limited by the fact that the supply of donor kidneys is small by comparison with the potential demand. In contrast to the demand for dialysis machines, which are abundantly available, competing demands for donor kidneys—among older and younger patients, or among any patients—raise an array of complicated ethical dilemmas involving issues of longevity, quality of life, and conflicting measures of social worth.

Data indicate, for example, that the survival of kidney transplant grafts among elderly recipients is at least 10 percent longer than that in younger patients. Moreover, younger patients (depending upon the diagnosis of the primary renal disease) do not necessarily have a markedly better prognosis for survival following transplantation than do older patients. These facts underscore the argument that the selection of kidney transplant recipients should be based on criteria other than age alone.

As long as donor organs remain in limited supply, however, one must consider whether kidney transplantation in the elderly represents a wise use of a scarce resource. To increase the donor pool substantially, it has been suggested that, contrary to existing practice, older donors be accepted, at ages comparable to those of older recipients (Brynger et al., 1986). Such a change in practice would require an extensive educational campaign aimed at the general public, and at primary care physicians as well. Even if such an expanded pool of donor organs should develop, the fact that older patients can benefit very well from kidney transplants would need to be more widely known among primary care physicians and kidney specialists so that they would, in fact, refer their older ESRD patients to kidney transplant teams.

Heart Transplantation

Even more remarkable than the recent experience with renal transplantation is that with cardiac transplantation (Hosenpud et al., 1990). As shown in Table 3.7, there were tremendous yearly increases during the 1980s in the number both of cardiac transplants and of transplant programs in the United States. Much of this increase occurred shortly after the clinical introduction of cyclosporine, in the early 1980s.

The results of cardiac transplantation are impressive. During the

Table 3.7
U.S. Experience with Cardiac Transplantation, 1981–1988: Number of
Transplants Performed and Number of Cardiac Transplant Programs

Year	Number of Transplants	Number of Transplant Programs
1981	62	8
1982	103	10
1983	172	12
1984	346	37
1985	719	71
1986	1,368	115
1987	1,438	123
1988	1,647	141

Source: R. W. Evans, Battelle Human Affairs Research Center, Seattle, Washington.

precyclosporine era (between 1968 and 1979), cardiac transplant recipients had an average one-year survival rate of 64 percent and a five-
year survival rate of 39 percent (Evans, 1989a). During the cyclosporine
era (from 1980 on), the survival rates showed marked improvement.
The one-year survival rate increased to 87 percent, and the five-year
survival rate to 53 percent (Starnes and Shumway, 1987). It is now
estimated that over 25 percent of all cardiac transplant recipients will
retain their transplanted organs for 10 years or longer (Evans et al.,
1984; Evans et al., 1986).

As these results have improved so considerably, some transplant
teams have begun to focus their attention on elderly transplant candidates. As a result, there is no longer a clear, recognized upper age limit
for cardiac transplantation (Carrier et al., 1986; Frazier et al., 1989;
Miller et al., 1988; Olivari et al., 1988).

Until recently, heart transplantation in patients over the age of 55
was rare, because of both the small supply of heart donors and physicians' fears concerning higher morbidity and mortality in older patients (Miller et al., 1988). However, data for U.S. patients only from
the Registry of the International Society for Heart Transplantation
(summarized in Table 3.8) indicate that there has been a dramatic
increase in the percentage and the number of patients who are at least
55 years old at the time of transplantation (Kaye, 1987). The percentage
of patients receiving transplants who were over age 55 increased from
3 percent of the total in 1984 to 25 percent in 1986.

The worldwide experience with cardiac transplantation provides
evidence of transplants at even older ages. As shown in Table 3.9, over
a 20-year period ending in 1988, 254 transplants, or 4.0 percent of
those performed, were in patients 60 years of age or older (Shumway

Table 3.8
Heart Transplant Recipients Older than 55 Years, in United States, 1973–1986

Years	Number of Recipients of All Ages	Recipients Older than 55 Years	
		Number	Percentage
1973–1983	555	13	2
1984	342	10	3
1985	671	98	15
1986	1003	249	25

Source: Miller et al., 1988, p. 254.

Table 3.9
Patients Who Received Heart Transplants, Worldwide, 1967 through September 25, 1988, by Age

Age (years)	Number of Patients	Age (years)	Number of Patients
0–04	74	35–39	641
5–09	45	40–44	932
10–14	120	45–49	1,176
15–19	218	50–54	1,182
20–24	308	55–59	768
25–29	322	60–64	230
30–34	384	65–69	24
		Total	6,424

Source: Shumway and Kaye, 1988, p. 2; with permission.

and Kaye, 1988). For the entire calendar year 1988, 2800 heart transplants were performed on persons aged 50 to 59 and 504 on persons aged 60 to 69; 41.3 percent of all cardiac transplants worldwide have been performed on persons 50 years of age and older. Morcover, 6.3 percent of cardiac transplants have been performed on persons 60 to 69 years of age (Hěck et al., 1989, p. 272).

Even though experience with cardiac transplantation in older persons is increasing, it is still quite limited. Two important studies have been published on the subject, however, which indicate that some older patients can be excellent candidates for transplant surgery.

One study (Miller et al., 1988) reports on 30 consecutive patients who underwent cardiac transplantation at Saint Louis University Hospital between May 1985 and October 1986. Eight of the 30 patients (the older group) were over age 55, with an average age of 57 at the time of transplantation; the oldest patient was aged 62. The other 22 patients (the younger group) were under age 55, with an average age of 38.2 years. The older group, generally, were in an advanced degree of heart failure at the time of transplantation; 5 of the 8 were confined to an intensive care unit, including 1 patient whose heart required a mechanical assistive device to sustain it until the transplantation could take place.

The results of the Saint Louis experience are as follows: four patients died, all of whom were in the younger group. Both groups tolerated cyclosporine therapy equally well, although many patients exhibited a variety of symptoms during the therapy. The older group experienced proportionately fewer episodes of treated transplant rejection than did the younger group. Following surgery, the incidence of infection per patient-month was similar in the groups. The 26 survivors in both groups were New York Heart Association (NYHA) class I—that is, near normal in cardiac function—within three months of transplantation, and all of the patients in the older group were gainfully employed; 6 of the 8 worked full-time.

In light of these findings, the authors of this study conclude that "patients over age 55 years can undergo transplantation with similar expectations as younger patients for survival, infection, rejection, nephrotoxicity, rehabilitation, and employability." They do, however, add a note of caution: "Care must be taken not to interpret these data as an endorsement of all patients of this age or older who might be candidates for a heart transplant, but we believe that it offers encouraging data for the carefully selected individual" (Miller et al., 1988, p. 257).

Another study, at the University of Minnesota, reported on 57 cardiac transplants performed in 1985 and 1986, including 23 in patients aged 55 to 65, who averaged 58 years of age (Olivari et al., 1988). In several important dimensions, the older patients fared as well as or better than the younger ones, who were between the ages of 6 months and 54 years. The probability of survival and the average rate of freedom from transplant rejection were identical in the two groups. Both had an average one-year survival rate of 96 percent, and 94 percent of patients in both groups were free of transplant rejection 12 months after surgery. The initial hospital stay averaged 13 days in the older group and 16 in the younger group. The mortality rate and the incidence of cerebrovascular accident during and/or immediately after surgery were similarly low in the two groups. However, the older group experienced higher rates of diabetes caused by drug therapy (17 percent versus 9 percent); and osteoporosis, also caused by drug therapy, was significantly higher in the older patients (13 percent versus 3 percent).

Although the incidence of infection was not significantly higher in the older patients than in the younger ones, life-threatening infection was observed only in the older patients. The rehabilitation status of the two patient groups also differed significantly, with 68 percent of the younger patients returning to work, compared with 35 percent of the older patients.

These findings led the Minnesota team to the following conclusions: "(1) heart transplantation is a valued therapeutic option even in elderly patients with end-stage heart failure, (2) it can be performed in selected patients at no increased operative risk with excellent long-term survival, (3) however, older patients are at high risk for serious infections and for developing steroid-related complications" (Olivari et al., 1988, p. 264). In particular, the authors state that patients with potential sources of infection, profound general deterioration due to heart disease, and evidence of generalized osteoporosis should be categorically excluded.

A consistent theme emerges from these two reports on cardiac transplantation in elderly persons: the selection of older patients must be handled with utmost care. While an elderly patient may benefit from cardiac transplantation, the experience with such patients has by no means been uniform. Simple guidelines are not available on the basis of the limited experience thus far.

It is probable that with increased experience the selection and care of the elderly cardiac transplant recipient can be further refined. However, due to a shortage of suitable donors and stiff competition for organs on behalf of younger transplant candidates, the accumulation of experience and knowledge in this area is likely to take considerable time and much effort. Moreover, the cost of cardiac transplantation remains a serious concern (Evans, 1986a; Evans, 1987a; Saywell et al., 1989). According to a recent report from the U.S. General Accounting Office (1989), based on 1987 data, the average charge for a cardiac transplant in the United States was $114,601. The average charge for the procedure in the 19 hospitals surveyed ranged from $51,829 to $121,330. Thus, much debate is certain to continue regarding the cost-effectiveness of cardiac transplantation, regardless of the age of the patient.

Older Patients and the Costs of Advanced Medical Technology

It is clear that advanced medical technologies such as dialysis, kidney transplantation, and heart transplantation are being used on behalf of older patients; and it is also clear that these older patients generally benefit to the same extent as do younger patients. The number of kidney and heart transplants in older persons could easily increase if larger supplies of donor organs were to develop. Undoubtedly, new advanced medical technologies will continue to be devised. Who or what will determine whether they are applied to older patients, or denied to them, and in what circumstances?

Medicare as a "Gatekeeper" for Advanced Technology

While Medicare is well known as a program that provides health insurance entitlements for older persons, the permanently disabled, and patients with ESRD, it is not as widely recognized for the critical role that it plays in the development, the application, and the diffusion of new medical technologies within the health care delivery system (Blumenthal et al., 1988; Mariano, 1989). For example, Medicare was the primary payer when the Jarvik total artificial heart was implanted into Seattle dentist Barney Clark. Although the implantation of the device was considered an experimental procedure and was therefore not reimbursed by Medicare, the subsequent care required by Clark was paid for by the Medicare program (Davis, 1985; Evans, in press). Additionally, a most notable decision was made several years ago when Medicare decided to pay for heart transplants but restricted eligibility to only those persons who met existing eligibility criteria (Evans, 1987b; Renlund et al., 1987). In other words, coverage was not extended to the entire population of the U.S. as was previously the case for persons in need of a kidney transplant or kidney dialysis.

Private health insurers look to the Medicare program for guidance on coverage determinations, decisions as to whether payment should be made for new and innovative medical technologies, and on reimbursement determinations, which set specific levels of acceptable payment for such procedures (Schaffarzick, 1987; Towery and Perry, 1981). In effect, Medicare coverage and reimbursement determinations are major societal mechanisms for allocating scarce health care resources. Denial of coverage by Medicare and restricted levels of reimbursement conserve Medicare expenditures, of course; but they also determine more generally which patients will have access to a new procedure, by indirectly limiting its availability to those patients who can pay for it out-of-pocket and/or to those who can afford a private insurance policy that will provide coverage (Evans, 1986b; Evans, 1989b).

Coverage determinations by Medicare for new medical and surgical procedures tend to focus on whether their efficacy is "questionable" and whether they are "cost-neutral" (that is, whether the cost of treating a patient with the new procedure is no greater than using an established treatment for the same medical condition). If a new drug, procedure, or treatment is cost-neutral, or nearly so, then approval of coverage by Medicare is usually straightforward. However, cost-neutrality is rarely achieved and is rarely confirmed by Medicare's official evaluations.

To date, the expenditures of the Medicare program have been primarily contained by limiting participation in the program through restrictions on patients' eligibility, and/or by limiting the extent of coverage available. Thus, arguments in favor of extending Medicare benefits to patients with AIDS, persons with end-stage cardiac disease, or patients with end-stage liver disease have been met with opposition. Similarly, efforts intended to expand coverage to various experimental or investigational procedures, including new treatments for advanced cancer, have been rejected by the administrators of the Medicare program.

Medicare and the Costs of Advanced Technology

Despite these and other efforts to contain the costs of the Medicare program, both enrollments and expenditures have increased steadily over the years. Between 1966 and 1987, as shown in Table 3.10, enrollment in the program increased by over 10 million people, much of the increase attributable to the increased number of eligible persons aged 65 and over in the American population (Mariano, 1989). Not surprisingly, the expenditures of the Medicare program have also increased notably. The total Medicare expenditure in 1970 was $7.5 billion, representing 0.8 percent of the gross national product (GNP) and 10.1 percent of all national health care expenditures (Table 3.11). By 1987, the total Medicare expenditure had increased more than tenfold, to $80.8 billion, or 1.8 percent of the GNP and 16.3 percent of the total national health care expenditure (Helbing and Keene, 1989).

Table 3.10
Number and Median Age of Medicare Enrollees and Percentage Distribution by Age, for Selected Years, 1966–1987

Year	Number of Enrollees	Median Age, All Enrollees	Percentage Distribution by Age (years)				
			65–69	70–74	75–79	80–84	85+
1966	19,108,822	72.8	34.2	28.7	19.7	11.2	6.2
1973	21,814,825	73.1	33.5	26.5	19.8	12.4	7.8
1980	25,515,070	73.2	33.1	26.4	18.9	12.2	9.4
1986	28,791,162	73.5	31.8	26.2	19.4	12.4	10.2
1987	29,380,480	73.5	31.8	26.0	19.4	12.6	10.3
Average annual increase (%)	2.1		1.7	1.6	2.0	2.6	4.6

Source: Mariano, 1989, p. 124.

Table 3.11
Medicare Expenditures for Selected Years, 1970–1987

Calendar Year	Amount (in billions)	Percentage of Gross National Product	Percentage of National Health Care Expenditures
1970	$ 7.5	0.8	10.1
1975	16.3	1.1	12.3
1980	36.8	1.3	14.9
1981	44.7	1.5	15.7
1982	52.4	1.7	16.3
1983	58.8	1.7	16.6
1984	64.6	1.7	16.7
1985	72.3	1.8	17.1
1986	77.7	1.8	17.0
1987	80.8	1.8	16.3

Source: Helbing and Keene, 1989, p. 111.

Table 3.12
National Health Care Expenditures for Selected Years, 1965–1987

Year	Amount (in billions)	Percentage of Gross National Product
1965	$ 41.9	5.9
1970	75.0	7.4
1975	132.7	8.3
1980	248.1	9.1
1981	287.0	9.4
1982	323.6	10.2
1983	357.2	10.5
1984	388.5	10.3
1985	419.0	10.4
1986	455.7	10.7
1987	500.3	11.1

Source: Levit et al., 1989, p. 3.

These increased Medicare expenditures in large part reflect the general growth of U.S. health care expenditures. As indicated in Table 3.12, national health care expenditures totaled $41.9 billion (or 5.9 percent of the GNP) in 1965, and by 1987 they had increased more than tenfold, to $500.3 billion (11.1 percent of the GNP). In 1990 these figures are expected to rise to $647.3 billion, or 12.0 percent of the GNP (Levit et al., 1989).

Even though the use of advanced medical technology is often criticized for contributing heavily to the escalation in health care expenditures (Callahan, 1987; Callahan, 1990; de Lissovoy, 1988; Lamm, 1989), few analysts have even attempted to evaluate the impact costly medical technologies have had on the Medicare program.

In evaluating the costs of medical technology, it is important to distinguish between two concepts, *procedure* (or treatment) *expenditures* and *program expenditures* (Evans, in press; Levit et al., 1989). The term *program expenditures* refers to the cumulative impact of the costs associated with all procedures performed or treatments provided. Thus, while individual procedures may be expensive, their economic impact is limited if the number of beneficiaries is small. Alternatively, program expenditures may be considerable if the procedure or treatment costs are low but the number of beneficiaries is large.

It is noteworthy that heart transplant coverage for Medicare beneficiaries, for instance, is projected to have relatively trivial implications for program expenditures. Because of a shortage of donor organs, as well as the use of strict criteria for patient selection, the Health Care Financing Administration projected a cost of $25.0 million for a probable 143 heart transplants in fiscal year 1991 (Roper, 1987). As this illustration suggests, expensive medical and surgical treatments need not have major consequences for program costs. The frequency with which a technology is likely to be used is an essential part of the equation.

The evidence is clear, however, that there has been a substantial increase in the number of complex surgical procedures performed on Medicare beneficiaries. For example, in 1972, 2,500 coronary artery bypass graft (CABG) procedures were performed on persons aged 65 to 74, and about 100 on persons aged 75 and over. By 1981, these figures had increased to 46,000 such procedures performed on persons aged 65 to 74 and 6,800 on persons aged 75 and older (Valvona and Sloan, 1985). More recent data from the National Center for Health Statistics (Kozak, 1989) indicate that the number of CABG procedures performed on persons aged 65 and over increased to 67,000 in 1983 and ballooned to 152,000 in 1987. At a cost in excess of $25,000 per procedure—even though actual Medicare reimbursements are somewhat less under its prospective payment system—it is apparent that CABG surgery has enormous implications for Medicare program expenditures.

The frequency of hip replacement surgery has also increased greatly over the past 17 years. In 1972, 25,000 procedures were performed on persons aged 65 and over, whereas by 1981 the comparable figure for that age group was 52,800 (Valvona and Sloan, 1985). Today, in the United States, the rate of total hip replacement, unadjusted for age and sex, is almost 309 operations per 100,000 persons (Liang et al., 1987), although older persons are the primary beneficiaries. The aggregate cost of total hip replacements in the United States was an estimated $690 million in 1979, and in 1985 it approached $4 billion. The average cost for a single, uncomplicated total hip replacement in one center in the United States averaged $23,000 in 1985. Clearly, as is the case with CABG surgery, the cost implications of total hip replacement for the Medicare program are substantial.

Based on the foregoing evidence, it is certainly reasonable to assume that advanced medical technology has directly contributed to the increase in the expenditures of the Medicare program. At the same time, we have seen in our review of experiences with kidney and heart transplantations performed on older persons that physicians have carefully selected for surgery only those older patients who are highly likely to benefit from these advanced procedures. There is nothing to suggest that Medicare, or health care expenditures generally, are wasted by applying advanced medical technologies to such older persons. In the final analysis, the advance of medical technology, itself, may have less drastic consequences for the expenditures of the Medicare program than will the increasingly large number of older patients who will be suitable candidates for the benefits of advanced technological intervention in the decades to come.

Balancing Costs and Benefits

As the Office of Technology Assessment concluded in its extensive report *Life-Sustaining Technologies and the Elderly*, "available data on the costs of life sustaining technologies are piecemeal and not comparable" (U.S. Congress, Office of Technology Assessment, 1987, p. 12). It must be added that the costs of advanced technology are only part of a much larger issue of costs and benefits.

In addition to economic costs, one must consider the benefits to the patients, to their families, to their friends, and to society. As we have seen from the technologies reviewed in this chapter, older patients benefit to the same extent as do younger patients (and perhaps to a greater extent, in terms of some broader, nonphysiological measures). Also, it may well be that patients who undergo advanced technological procedures benefit from a much higher quality of life than they would otherwise have experienced.

Even with respect to economic costs, no proper assessment can be made without making a comparison between the price of performing a sophisticated technological intervention, and the health care dollars that would likely be expended on that patient if the advanced procedure were not performed. As we have seen in this chapter, the costs of providing a kidney transplant and associated treatment to a patient who survives and benefits for several years can be less than the costs of providing kidney dialysis over the same period. More generally, comparisons need to be made between the costs of using high technology that can enable older patients to regain independent functional capacity in the activities of daily living, and the costs of providing long-term care to those same patients (see Scitovsky, 1988)—in nursing homes, or through services in other domiciliary arrangements—which may compound in total expenditures through years of dependency.

There are also the in-kind and indirect costs involved in sustaining a chronically ill or disabled person who does not receive the benefits of advanced medical technology. For some time it has been well established that family care of dependent older persons is pervasive in our society, and that families (rather than formal service systems) provide 80 to 90 percent of medically related and personal care, as well as assistance in household tasks, transportation, and shopping, to disabled older persons who are not in nursing homes (Brody, 1985; U.S. Senate, Special Committee on Aging, 1985). The physical, psychological, familial, and social burdens on these family caregivers are becoming well documented (Chappell, 1990); and programs designed and funded to relieve their burdens (e.g., "adult day care" and "respite" programs) have begun to proliferate throughout the nation. The nonmonetary costs of family burdens and the monetary costs of the programs that help to relieve these burdens must also be included in the equation that attempts to evaluate the relative expense of treating older persons through advanced medical technology.

These complex issues of costs and benefits make it extremely difficult to balance patients' needs with the constraints of limited resources for providing treatment. Especially in a context of scarcity—as is the case with donor organs, as discussed in this chapter—it is easy to be tempted to use chronological age as a relatively simple criterion for determining access to medical care. However, as we have seen, old age is not necessarily an important predictor of outcome. Arguments regarding the costs to society of using advanced medical technology are not overwhelmingly persuasive when applied to older persons.

Chronic debilitating disease will become more prevalent as our population continues to age. As advanced medical technologies continue to evolve, we will increasingly face a greater number of complicated therapeutic and policy decisions that will affect the length and the quality of older persons' lives. Inevitably, questions will recur regarding the wisdom of allocating limited health resources to the aged (Battin, 1987).

At the same time, it is apparent that older persons will continue to fulfill a useful role in our society, and that they should not be denied the opportunity to do so solely on the basis of their chronological age. To bar older persons from access to medical advances achieved during their lifetimes would seem to be a particularly unfitting conclusion to their lives, and a profound indictment of the society in which we live. How we eventually deal with the issues of allocating new medical technologies to the aged will tell us a great deal about how people are valued, generally, in our society.

Appendix: The Life Expectancy and Aging of the United States Population, and the Prevalance of Chronic Disease and Morbidity at Older Ages

Table A.1
U.S. Life Expectancy at Birth, by Gender, 1940–1986

Year	Both Sexes	Male	Female
1986	74.8	71.3	78.3
1985	74.7	71.2	78.2
1984	74.7	71.2	78.2
1983	74.6	71.0	78.1
1982	74.5	70.9	78.1
1981	74.2	70.4	77.8
1980	73.7	70.0	77.4
1979	73.9	70.0	77.8
1978	73.5	69.6	77.3
1977	73.3	69.5	77.2
1976	72.9	69.1	76.8
1975	72.6	68.8	76.6
1974	72.0	68.2	75.9
1973	71.4	67.6	75.3
1972	71.2	67.4	75.1
1971	71.1	67.4	75.0
1970	70.8	67.1	74.7
1960	69.7	66.6	73.1
1950	68.2	65.6	71.1
1940	62.9	60.8	65.2

Source: National Center for Health Statistics (1988). Advance report of final mortality statistics, 1986. *Monthly Vital Statistics Report*, vol. 37, no. 6, suppl. DHHS Pub. no. (PHS) 88-1120. Hyattsville, Md.: U.S. Public Health Service.

Table A.2
Percentage of U.S. Population in Older Age Groups, 1950–2020

Age Group	Actual Percentage				Middle Series Projection of Percentage, 1985–2020				
	1950	*1960*	*1970*	*1980*	*1985*	*1990*	*2000*	*2010*	*2020*
60 and over	12.1	13.2	14.1	15.7	16.6	17.0	17.0	19.5	24.0
65 and over	8.1	9.3	9.9	11.3	12.0	12.7	13.1	13.9	17.3
70 and over	4.8	5.8	6.4	7.4	8.1	8.7	9.7	9.7	11.7
75 and over	2.6	3.1	3.7	4.4	4.9	5.5	6.5	6.7	7.3
80 and over	1.1	1.4	1.8	2.3	2.6	3.0	3.8	4.3	4.4
85 and over	0.4	0.5	0.7	1.0	1.2	1.4	1.9	2.4	2.5

Source: U.S. Bureau of the Census (1984). Demographic and socioeconomic aspects of aging in the United States. *Current Population Reports*, ser. P-23, no. 138, p. 17. Washington, D.C.: U.S. Government Printing Office.

Table A.3
Prevalence of Nine Chronic Conditions in U.S. Population Aged 60 and Over

Condition	Percent of Population Aged 60 and Over
Arthritis	49.0
Hypertension	41.8
Cataracts	19.9
Heart disease	14.0
Varicose veins	9.9
Diabetes	9.5
Cancer (except nonmelanoma skin cancer)	6.6
Osteoporosis or hip fracture	5.5
Stroke	5.4

Source: Guralnik, La Croix, Everett, and Kovar (1989). Aging in the eighties: the prevalence of comorbidity and its association with disability. *Advance Data from Vital and Health Statistics*, no. 170. Hyattsville, Md.: National Center for Health Statistics.

Table A.4
Percentage of Persons in Older Age Groups with No, One, and Two or More Chronic Conditions, by Gender, 1984

Age (years)	Number of Chronic Conditions		
	0	1	2 or More
Men			
60–69	30	35	35
70–79	22	31	47
≥80	19	28	53
Women			
60–69	23	32	45
70–79	14	25	61
≥80	10	20	70

Source: Guralnik, La Croix, Everett, and Kovar (1989). Aging in the eighties: the prevalence of comorbidity and its association with disability. *Advance Data from Vital and Health Statistics*, no. 170. Hyattsville, Md.: National Center for Health Statistics.

Table A.5
Percentage of Persons, by Older Age Groups and Gender, Having Difficulty with One or More Activities of Daily Living, United States, 1984

Age (years)	Number of Activities					
	0	1	2	3	4	5
Men						
60–69	3.6	8.9	16.9	30.4	50.4	45.2
70–79	5.2	12.5	21.1	31.2	48.7	59.9
≥80	13.3	29.2	36.6	32.7	51.5	87.0
Women						
60–69	3.0	10.5	17.0	26.8	33.9	60.6
70–79	5.2	14.7	22.6	33.3	47.1	58.4
≥80	14.0	24.4	38.8	52.0	66.9	79.2

Source: Guralnik, La Croix, Everett, and Kovar (1989). Aging in the eighties: the prevalence of comorbidity and its association with disability. *Advance Data from Vital and Health Statistics*, no. 170. Hyattsville, Md.: National Center for Health Statistics.

References

Aaron, H.J., and Schwartz, W.B. (1984). *The painful prescription: rationing hospital care.* Washington, D.C.: Brookings Institution.

Avorn, J. (1984). Benefit and cost analysis in geriatric care: turning age discrimination into health policy. *New England Journal of Medicine, 310*, 1294–1301.

Battin, M.P. (1987). Is there a duty to die? *Ethics, 97*(2), 317–340.

Birren, J.E. (1986). The process of aging: growing up and growing old. In A. Pifer and L. Bronte, eds., *Our changing society: paradox and promise*, pp. 263–281. New York: W.W. Norton.

Blumenthal, D., Schlesinger, M., and Drumheller, P.B. (1988). *Renewing the promise: Medicare and its reform.* New York: Oxford University Press.

Brody, E.M. (1985). Parent care as a normative family stress. *Gerontologist, 25*, 19–29.

Brynger, H., Persson, H., and Blohme, I. (1986). Renal transplantation in elderly patients. *Transplantation Proceedings, 18*(suppl. 3), 12–13.

Callahan, D. (1987). *Setting limits: medical goals in an aging society.* New York: Simon & Schuster.

Callahan, D. (1988). Allocating health resources. *Hastings Center Report, 18*(2), 1420.

Callahan, D. (1989). Old age and new policy. *Journal of the American Medical Association, 261*, 905–906.

Callahan, D. (1990). *What kind of life: the limits of medical progress.* New York: Simon & Schuster.

Canadian Transplant Study Group (1985). Examination of parameters influencing the benefit:detriment ratio of cyclosporine in renal transplantation. *American Journal of Kidney Diseases, 5*, 328–332.

Cardella, C.J., Harding, M.E., Abraham, G., Robinson, C., Oreopoulos, D., Uldall, P.R., Jordan, M., Cook, G., Struthers, N., Honery, R., Bear, R., and Cole, E. (1989). Renal transplantation in older patients on peritoneal dialysis. *Transplantation Proceedings, 21*(1), 2022–2023.

Carrier, M., Emery, R.W., Riley, J.E., Levinson, M.M., and Copeland, J.G. (1986). Cardiac transplantation in patients over 50 years of age. *Journal of the American College of Cardiology, 8*, 285–288.

Castro, L.A. (1986). Indications for renal transplantation. *Transplantation Proceedings, 18*(suppl. 3), 5–7.

Chappell, N.L. (1990). Aging and social care. In R.H. Binstock and L.K. George, eds., *Handbook of aging and the social sciences* (3rd edition), pp. 438–454. San Diego, Calif.: Academic Press.

Colen, B.D. (1986). *Hard choices: mixed blessings of modern medical technology.* New York: G.P. Putnam's Sons.

Daniels, N. (1987). *Am I my parent's keeper? an essay on justice between the young and the old.* New York: Oxford University Press.

Davis, C.K. (1985). The impact of prospective payment on clinical research. *Journal of the American Medical Association, 253*, 686–687.

de Lissovoy, G. (1988). Medicare and heart transplants. *Health Affairs*, 7(4), 61–72.

Edmunds, L.H., Stephenson, L.W., Edie, R.N., and Ratcliffe, M.B. (1988). Open-heart surgery in octogenarians. *New England Journal of Medicine*, 319, 131–136.

Eggers, P.W. (1988). Effect of transplantation on the Medicare end-stage renal disease program. *New England Journal of Medicine*, 318, 223–229.

Evans, R.W. (1986a). Cost-effectiveness analysis of transplantation. *Surgical Clinics of North America*, 66(3), 603–616.

Evans, R.W. (1986b). Coverage and reimbursement for heart transplantation. *International Journal of Technology Assessment in Health Care*, 2, 425–429.

Evans, R.W. (1987a). The economics of heart transplantation. *Circulation*, 75(1), 63–67.

Evans, R.W. (1987b). Medicare-designated centers for cardiac transplantation. *New England Journal of Medicine*, 317, 966.

Evans, R.W. (1989a). *The failures of success in organ transplantation*. Seattle, Wash.: Battelle Human Affairs Research Centers.

Evans, R.W. (1989b). Money matters: should ability to pay ever be a consideration in gaining access to transplantation? *Transplantation Proceedings*, 21(3), 3419–3423.

Evans, R.W. (1990). Organ donation: new ways needed to keep up with demand, part 2. *Nephrology News and Issues*, 4(6), 14–15.

Evans, R.W. (in press). Xenotransplantation: a panel discussion of some nonclinical issues. In M.A. Hardy, ed., *Xenograft 25*. Amsterdam: Elsevier Science Publishing.

Evans, R.W., Blagg, C.R., and Bryan, F.A., Jr. (1981). Implications for health care policy: a social and demographic profile of hemodialysis in the United States. *Journal of the American Medical Association*, 245, 487–491.

Evans, R.W., Manninen, D.L., Garrison, L.P., Jr., and Hart, L.G. (1987). *Special report: findings from the national kidney dialysis and kidney transplantation study*. HCFA Pub. no. 03230. Baltimore, Md.: Health Care Financing Administration.

Evans, R.W., Manninen, D.L., Garrison, L.P., Jr., Hart, L.G., Blagg, C.R., Gutman, R.A., Hull, A.R., and Lowrie, E.G. (1985). The quality of life of patients with end-stage renal disease. *New England Journal of Medicine*, 312, 553–559.

Evans, R.W., Manninen, D.L., Garrison, L.P., Jr., and Maier, A. (1986). Donor availability as the primary determinant of the future of heart transplantation. *Journal of the American Medical Association*, 255, 1892–1898.

Evans, R.W., Manninen, D.L., Overcast, T.D., Garrison, L.P., Jr., Yagi, J., Merrikin, K., and Jonsen, A.R. (1984). *The national heart transplantation study: final report*. Seattle, Wash.: Battelle Human Affairs Research Centers.

Evans, R.W., Manninen, D.L., and Thompson, C. (1989). *A cost and outcome analysis of kidney transplantation: the implications of initial immunosuppressive protocol and diabetes*. Seattle, Wash.: Battelle Human Affairs Research Centers.

Fehrman, I., Brattstrom, C., Duraj, F., and Groth, C.G. (1989). Kidney transplantation in patients between 65 and 75 years of age. *Transplantation Proceedings, 21*(1), 2018–2019.

Frazier, O.H., Macris, M.P., Lammermeier, D.E., Duncan, J.M., Radovancevik, B., and Van Buren, C.T. (1989). Heart transplantation in 234 patients: review of the Texas Heart Institute six-year experience. *Transplantation Proceedings, 21*(1), 2489.

Fryd, D.S., So, S.K.S., Kruse, L., Seifeldin, R., Canafax, D.M., Sutherland, D.E.R., Simmons, R.L., and Najarian, J.S. (1987). Improving results of renal transplantation with multidrug therapy in patients over 50 years of age. *Clinical Transplantation, 1*, 75–80.

Gordon, R.D., Starzl, T.E., Hakala, T.R., Taylor, R.J., Schroter, G.P.J., Rosenthal, J.T., Weil, R., III, Iwatsuki, S., and Carpenter, B.J. (1987). Long-term results of cyclosporine-steroid therapy in 131 nonmatched cadaveric renal transplants. *Clinical Transplantation, 1*, 44–48.

Health Care Financing Administration (1988). *Research report: end-stage renal disease, 1986.* HCFA pub. no. 03268. Baltimore, Md.: Health Care Financing Administration.

Health Care Financing Administration (1989). *Research report: end-state renal disease, 1987.* HCFA pub. no. 03288. Baltimore, Md.: Health Care Financing Administration.

Heck, C.F., Shumway, S.J., and Kaye, M.P. (1989). The registry of the International Society for Heart Transplantation: sixth official report. *Journal of Heart Transplantation, 8*, 271–276.

Helbing, C., and Keene, R. (1989). Use and cost of physician and supplier services under Medicare, 1986. *Health Care Financing Review, 10*(3), 109–122.

Hosenpud, J.D., Pantely, G.A., Norman, D.J. Cobanoglu, A.M., Hovaguimian, H., and Starr, A. (1990). A critical analysis of morbidity and mortality as it relates to recipient age following cardiac transplantation. *Clinical Transplantation, 4*, 51–54.

Howard, R.J., Pfaff, W.W., Salomon, D., Peterson, J., Scornik, J.C., Frederickson, E., and Fennell, R.S., III (1989). Kidney transplantation in older patients. *Transplantation Proceedings, 21*(1), 2020–2021.

Ito, T., Iwaki, Y., and Terasaki, P.I. (1986). Donor and recipient age effect. In P.I. Terasaki, ed., *Clinical transplants, 1986,* pp. 189–197. Los Angeles: UCLA Tissue Typing Laboratory.

Kaye, M.P. (1987). The Registry of the International Society for Heart Transplantation: fourth official report—1987. *Journal of Heart Transplantation, 6*, 63–67.

Kock, B., Kuhlback, B., Ahonen, J., Lindfors, O., and Lindstrom, B.L. (1980). Kidney transplantation in patients over 60 years of age. *Scandinavian Journal of Urology and Nephrology, 54*(suppl.), 103–105.

Kozak, L.J. (1989). Hospital inpatient surgery: United States, 1983–87. *Vital and Health Statistics,* no. 169. DHHS Pub. no. (PHS) 89-1250. Hyattsville, Md.: U.S. Public Health Service, National Center for Health Statistics.

Lamm, R.D. (1989). Saving a few, sacrificing many—at great cost. *New York Times*, August 2, p. 28.

Lauffer, G., Murie, J.A., Gray, D., Ting, A., and Morris, P.J. (1988). Renal transplantation in patients over 55 years old. *British Journal of Surgery, 75*, 984–987.

Levit, K.R., Freeland, M.S., and Waldo, D.R. (1989). Health spending and ability to pay: business, individuals, and government. *Health Care Financing Review, 10*(3), 1–11.

Liang, M.H., Wade, J., Hartley, R.M., Cullen, K.E., and Caplan, A.L. (1987). Social and health policy issues in total joint replacement therapy. *International Journal of Technology Assessment, 3*, 387–395.

Lowance, D.C. (1988). Withdrawal from dialysis: an ethical perspective. *Kidney International, 34*, 124–135.

Mailloux, L.U., Bellucci, A.G., and Mossey, R.T. (1988). Predictors of survival in patients undergoing dialysis. *American Journal of Medicine, 84*, 855–862.

Mariano, L.A. (1989). Growth in the Medicare population. *Health Care Financing Review, 10*(3), 123–124.

Mauer, S.M., Caplan, A., Nevins, T.E., and Najarian, J.S. (1989). Renal transplantation for children. *Journal of the American Medical Association, 262*, 348.

Miller, L.W., Vitale-Noedel, N., Pennington, G., McBride, L., and Kanter, K.R. (1988). Heart transplantation in patients over age fifty-five years. *Journal of Heart/Transplantation, 7*, 254–257.

Moskop, J.C. (1987). The moral limits to federal funding for kidney disease. *Hastings Center Report, 17*(2), 11–15.

Murie, J.A., Lauffer, G., Gray, D., Ting, A., and Morris, P.J. (1989). Renal transplantation in the older patient. *Transplantation Proceedings, 21*(1), 2024–2025.

Neu, S.C., and Kjellstrand, C. (1986). Stopping long-term dialysis: an empirical study of withdrawal of life supporting treatment. *New England Journal of Medicine, 314*, 14–20.

Offner, G., Pichlmayr, R., Hoyer, P.T., Buzendahl, H., Ringe, B., Wonigeit, K., and Brodehl, J. (1989). Renal transplantation in pediatric patients with special reference to long-term cyclosporin treatment in childhood. *Clinical Transplantation, 3*, 75–77.

Olivari, M.T., Antolick, A., Kaye, M.P., Jamieson, S.W., and Ring, W.S. (1988). Heart transplantation in elderly patients. *Journal of Heart Transplantation, 7*, 258–264.

Ost, L., Groth, C.G., Lindholm, B., Lundgren, G., Magnusson, G., and Tillegard, A. (1980). Cadaveric renal transplantation in patients of 60 years and above. *Transplantation, 30*, 339.

Pirsch, J.D., Stratta, R.J., Armbrust, M.J., D'Allessandro, A.M., Sollinger, H.W., Kalayoglu, M., and Belzer, F.O. (1989). Cadaveric renal transplantation with cyclosporine in patients more than 60 years of age. *Transplantation, 47*, 259–261.

Renlund, D.G., Bristow, M.R., Lybert, M.R., O'Connell, J.B., and Gay, W.A.,

Jr. (1987). Medicare-designated centers for cardiac transplantation. *New England Journal of Medicine, 316,* 873–876.

Roper, W.L. (1987). Medicare program: criteria for Medicare coverage of heart transplants. *Federal Register, 52*(65), 10935–10951.

Saywell, R.M., Jr., Woods, J.R., Halbrook, H.G., Jay, S.J., Nyhuis, A.S., and Lohrman, R.G. (1989). Cost analyses of heart transplantation from day of operation to the day of discharge. *Journal of Heart Transplantation, 8*(3), 244–252.

Schaffarzick, R.W. (1987). Technology assessment: perspective of a third-party payer. In K.N. Lohn and R.A. Rettig, eds., *Quality of care and technology assessment,* pp. 98–105. Washington, D.C.: Institute of Medicine, National Academy Press.

Schneider, E.L. (1989). Options to control the rising health care costs of older Americans. *Journal of the American Medical Association, 261,* 907–908.

Schwartz, W.B., and Aaron, H.J. (1984). Rationing hospital care: lessons from Britain. *New England Journal of Medicine, 310,* 52–56.

Scitovsky, A.A. (1988). Medical care in the last twelve months of life: age, functional status, and medical care expenditures. *Milbank Memorial Fund Quarterly/Health and Society, 66,* 640–660.

Shah, B., First, M.R., Munda, R., Penn, I., Fidler, J.P., and Alexander, J.W. (1988). Current experience with renal transplantation in older patients. *American Journal of Kidney Diseases, 12,* 516–523.

Shumway, S., and Kaye, M.P. (1988). The International Society for Heart Transplantation Registry. In P.I. Terasaki ed., *Clinical transplants, 1988,* pp. 1–4. Los Angeles: UCLA Tissue Typing Laboratory.

Starnes, V.A., and Shumway, N.E. (1987). Heart transplantation—Stanford experience. In P.I. Terasaki, ed., *Clinical transplants, 1987,* pp. 277–285. Los Angeles: UCLA Tissue Typing Laboratory.

Towery, O.B., and Perry, S. (1981). The scientific basis for coverage decisions by third-party payers. *Journal of the American Medical Association, 245,* 59–61.

U.S. Congress, Office of Technology Assessment (1987). *Life-sustaining technologies and the elderly.* Washington, D.C.: U.S. Government Printing Office.

U.S. General Accounting Office (1989). *Heart transplants: concerns about cost, access, and availability of donor organs.* GAO/HRD-89-61. Washington, D.C.: General Accounting Office.

U.S. Senate, Special Committee on Aging (1985). *America in transition: an aging society, 1984–85 edition.* Washington, D.C.: U.S. Government Printing Office.

Valvona, J., and Sloan, F. (1985). Rising rates of surgery among the elderly. *Health Affairs, 4*(3), 108–118.

Wedel, N., Brynger, H., and Blohme, I. (1980). Kidney transplantation in patients 60 years and older. *Scandinavian Journal of Urology and Nephrology 54*(suppl.), 106–108.

4

The Goals of Medicine in an Aging Society

CHRISTINE K. CASSEL, M.D., and
BERNICE L. NEUGARTEN, Ph.D.

The unprecedented aging of our society has recently set off a vigorous debate about the appropriate use of expensive and extensive medical care for elderly persons. This debate involves very complex issues, which are too often and too easily oversimplified both in the media and in the professional literature. Some argue that because the increases in longevity in the past two decades are largely the result of advances in medical technology, we can and should continue, by means of research and the implementation of new technologies, to push back the age barriers that presently create limits to good health and to length of life (e.g., Schneider, 1989). Others argue that there must be a natural end to the human life span, that old age is a reasonable and acceptable indicator of proximity to death, and that it is both unseemly and wasteful to keep augmenting medical technology in a struggle against the inevitability of death (e.g., Callahan, 1987).

In this chapter we will examine the goals of medicine in light of the dramatic demographic and epidemiologic changes in our society. We do this in the hope of developing a framework within which the complex questions about appropriate medical care for patients of advanced age can be addressed most rationally, most effectively, and most humanely.

The "State" of Modern Medicine

The decade of the 1970s saw the beginning of a reexamination of modern medicine. Many different and often conflicting voices were heard, as is true to the present day. Critics included John Knowles

75

(1977), who edited an issue of the journal *Daedalus* entitled *Doing Better and Feeling Worse*. The title referred to the apparent difference between objective indicators of health, which showed improvement; and subjective reports from patients, which indicated increases in health-related complaints as well as growing dissatisfaction with physicians and hospitals.

Carlson's book *The End of Medicine* (1975) also was an indication of the introspection going on in the medical profession and the public examination of the practice of medicine and its role in our society. The title of the book suggested both a critique of the end(s), or the goal(s), of medicine, and a prediction that an oversized technocracy that has outgrown its human roots must inevitably decline and come to an end. Similar apocalyptic visions were popularized by Ivan Illich in his book *Medical Nemesis* (1976), which put forward the view of modern medicine as too narrowly focused on reductionist technical approaches to problems that would be better approached through social reforms or preventive practices. Howard Waitzkin, in *The Second Sickness* (1983), argued that perverse financial incentives were responsible for the imbalances described by Illich, Carlson, and others.

This reexamination of the goals of medicine and the proper place of medicine in society continued through the 1980s, but the themes became more focused. In the 1970s attention was concentrated on the role that unbridled technology has played in diminishing the humanism of medicine. In the 1980s, it was focused on the costs of that technology and on the ways to stem the steadily increasing expenditures (see Hiatt, 1987).

Today, increasing costs are often described as being closely linked to the increase in life expectancy, because older people use far greater amounts of medical care than do younger people. The increasing life expectancy of Americans is, at least in part, due to advances in medical care. Moreover, because today people seldom die prematurely, they need more medical care to help cope with the chronic diseases of senescence. The special interplay between advanced medical technologies and increasing life expectancy has led to even greater questioning of the goals of medicine. The issues of cost containment and the risks of dehumanized technology are often invoked to argue for setting limits on the use of medical interventions, especially for aged persons (e.g., Callahan 1987; Callahan, 1990).

The goals of medicine in today's society must be examined in the context of medical technology and the rising costs of health care. Also, however, they must be reconsidered in light of the increasing longevity of the population, and the moral and ethical issues that underlie the practice of medicine.

The Increase in Life Expectancy

Longevity has increased dramatically in this century, with average life expectancy almost doubling in the period from 1900 to 1965. During that period, two basic assumptions were made. The first was that most of the decline in mortality was due to advances in social conditions rather than to advances in medical treatment. Better sanitation, nutrition, education, and working conditions were largely responsible for the drop in premature deaths that occurred, historically, long before the advent of any specific life-saving medical discoveries, such as insulin or antibiotics.

The second assumption was that the genetically determined life span of the human species is probably about 75 years. It was recognized that a gap exists between maximum life span and average length of life. By the mid-1960s, however, as average life expectancy began to approach 70 years, it was assumed that the gap had been narrowed about as much as possible: that, in short, we had come close to maximizing life expectancy in this country.

Within a decade, however, the latter assumption was proved wrong, and the great demographic transition of the 1980s had begun. Life expectancy, after remaining stable for two decades, began to increase again. This transition has been described in extraordinary detail by demographers, epidemiologists, and health policy specialists (e.g., Olshansky and Ault, 1986).

The increase in longevity has not yet reached a plateau, nor has it ended. In fact, it is continuing at an unprecedented and unanticipated rate. Average life expectancy is now nearly 80 years for women and nearly 74 years for men, and mortality rates are declining most rapidly among the persons who are over 85. The latter group presently constitutes about 1 percent of the population, but it is projected to be over 2 percent in the next 20 years (U.S. Senate, Special Committee on Aging, et al., 1987). While still a small percentage, the numbers of people in this age group, now some 5 million, will increase to as many as 20 million in two decades. A sense of how dramatic this phenomenon has been can be seen in the U.S. Bureau of the Census publication *The Centenarians* (1988), which describes the growth in the number of persons over the age of 100, a number that jumped from 15,000 in 1980 to 25,000 only five years later, in 1985. At that rate, it is predicted that the number will reach 110,000 by the year 2000 and will perhaps be tripled 30 years later, in 2030.

The recent sharp increase in life expectancy is probably due much more to advances in medical treatment than was the increase seen before the mid-1960s. It is difficult to explain the latest gains as the reflection of new social advances, and even more difficult to imagine that a genetic or other biological change has occurred in the human species that would account for such a dramatic demographic transition in a period of only two decades. Instead, the single major factor often described is the decline in mortality from cardiovascular disease which has occurred in the past 20 years. There is some evidence to support the idea that preventive health measures, combined with advanced medical treatment, are probably responsible for the fact that the onset of severe or potentially fatal coronary disease now occurs at a much later age than it did 10 to 15 years ago. Clearly enough, more research is needed to identify the factors contributing to the drop in mortality rates.

Added Longevity: Good or Bad?

The gain in longevity among Americans has been a remarkable phenomenon, and it is probably the mark of an advanced industrialized civilization, for it has also appeared in other industrialized countries of the world. But is it a good thing? Are we to be pleased that people are living so much longer than we ever thought they would? How we answer such questions has a great deal to do with our understanding of society's response to the demographic transition, and it relates directly to the basic issue of the goals of medicine in an aging society.

One way of looking at the issue is by asking, as people reach such advanced old age, how healthy and happy are they? Today, the majority of persons over 65 report at least one chronic illness. Reported illness and impairment, however, do not necessarily result in disability. It is the number and the severity of functional disabilities that are the preferred measures of health status. Persons consider themselves in ill health primarily when an illness or impairment interferes with their activities of daily living, usually defined as the tasks related to personal care and to maintenance of the home environment. As might be anticipated, such health-related difficulties increase with advancing age, yet it is noteworthy that of persons aged 65 to 74, the most recent data show that more than 80 percent report no limitations in carrying out these daily activities. Of those aged 75 to 84, more than 70 percent report no such limitations, and even of those over age 85, half report no limitations (U.S. Senate, Special Committee on Aging, et al., 1987).

This is not to underestimate the problems of those persons who are significantly burdened by ill health or those who are dependent on others for their day-to-day care. It is instead to point out that only a minority of older persons, even at advanced older ages, are ill or disabled. National surveys have also found repeatedly that older people report high levels of life satisfaction, as high as or sometimes higher than the levels reported by younger people (Campbell et al., 1976; Harris et al., 1975; Harris et al., 1981).

Not only are old people as a group faring well, but of at least equal importance in the present context is the fact that, as individuals, people. grow old in very different ways, and they become increasingly different from one another with the passage of years. Women age differently from men, and there are differences among racial, ethnic, and particularly, socioeconomic groups. Added to this are the idiosyncratic sequences of events that accumulate over lifetimes to create increasing individual variation. The result is that older people are a very diverse group.

Although the prevalence of illness and disability increases with age in the second half of life, the association between age and health is far from perfect. Age is a good predictor of health status in statistical terms, but for any given individual, age is a poor predictor of physical, mental, or social competence. This finding has emerged repeatedly in systematic studies of performance in which a wide range of physiologic and psychological variables has been examined (Shock et al., 1984) and has come to be called a "superfact" in gerontological research (Maddox, 1986; see also chapter 2 of this book).

The most optimistic analysts, exemplified by Fries (1980), predict that the overall health status of the elderly population will continue to improve, leading to a "compression of morbidity" in the last period of life. Others, exemplified by Brody and Schneider (1983), argue that an increase in life expectancy will lead to an increase in the average period of morbidity and dependency before death.

Recent studies that examine "active life expectancy" (e.g., Katz et al., 1983) attempt to forecast patterns of morbidity and disability, as well as length of life. In these studies, it appears that with advancing age, an increasing percentage of the remaining years of life is likely to be spent in a dependent or disabled state. For example, for persons who reach age 65, an average of 16.5 years of life remain. The forecast is that this period of 16-plus years will include, on average, 6 years (or 40 percent) spent in a state of disability and dependency. For persons who reach 85, it is projected that 7.5 years of life remain, a period that includes more than 4.5 years (or 60 percent) in a disabled state. These data support the prediction that the added years of life will be characterized by disability and dependency, and contradict the optimistic view that, as Fries predicts, most persons will stay healthy until about age 85, then die quickly.

It is the specter of disability, particularly mental impairment from chronic dementing diseases such as Alzheimer's disease, that is most frightening for older people and their families. Disability also creates the greatest need for long-term care, either in institutional or home settings. Alzheimer's disease, hip fracture, and other disorders that result in major loss of function increase exponentially after approximately age 75 to 80 (see Hing, 1987; Kane and Kane, 1990; Manton, 1990). This would suggest to some observers that it may be inappropriate to provide life-extending medical care to individuals in their late seventies or older if the life that is extended is simply a life of disability and dependency. These averages, however, do not adequately describe the tremendous physiologic, psychological, and social variability among members of any age cohort, as mentioned above.

Health Care Costs and the Appropriateness of Treatment

Many factors are contributing to the rise in health care costs, including general inflation, the rapid escalation of physicians' fees, and the mushrooming costs of hospital care, as well as the increase in the number of old people, with their needs for health care (see chapter 2, above). In this connection, it is important to note that a small proportion of older people, about 17 percent, account for over 60 percent of Medicare payments. This statistic confirms the fact that it is only a small fraction of older persons in any one year who are responsible of the high usage of medical services. It also is consistent with the observation that most old people are not very sick until the last year of their lives. One study showed that the 6 percent of Medicare beneficiaries who died during the year 1978 accounted for 28 percent of Medicare reimbursements in that year (Lubitz and Prihoda, 1984). Other studies of high-cost Medicare patients have shown that a considerable fraction of hospital costs are attributable to patients who die during their hospitalization or shortly after discharge (Scitovsky, 1984).

Such data have led to overly simplistic exhortations that old people, instead of irresponsibly consuming all these medical resources, should accept death and thus allow more resources to be used for the young (Callahan, 1987; Callahan, 1990; Lamm, 1987). Some commentators argue that investment in acute health care yields more potential years of life in the young than in the old, and thus it is a more prudential investment plan for society's health care dollars (Daniels, 1988).

Such statements raise fundamental moral questions about the value of human life. They also make misleading generalizations about the goals of most medical treatment, describing it as "life extension" rather than as providing comfort to the patient or enhancing the patient's functional status and quality of life. Just as it is difficult to generalize about the health status of "the elderly," it is equally difficult to generalize about the appropriate use of "medical technology." When the specific uses of the resources spent on patients in their last year of life are examined, it becomes clear that most such patients were functioning at a high level prior to their last illness. Furthermore, the large expenditures in the last year of life are much more likely to be for persons aged 65 to 80 than for persons aged 80 and over (Scitovsky, 1984).

In addition, physicians cannot predict at the onset of hospitalization which patients are likely to survive. As studies have suggested, half of the high-cost patients survive at reasonable levels of functional status for a year or more (Scitovsky, 1984). In other words, the high-cost Medicare patient has a 50:50 chance of meaningful survival. It would be difficult, on grounds of morality, to argue that for reasons of economy, not for medical reasons, all such patients should be allowed to die.

A basic question about the goals of medicine arises here. Persons in danger of dying are, by definition, persons who are extremely ill and are therefore likely to need extensive and expensive hospital care. It is not enough to look simply at the expenditures incurred for them; it may be quite appropriate to provide extensive hospital care for a person with a serious illness, especially if there is a reasonable likelihood of a successful outcome and if such care is consistent with the patient's values or expressed preferences.

The number of dollars spent does not necessarily reflect the appropriateness of any given medical intervention selected by the patient's physician. There is no doubt that life-extending technologies are sometimes used in treating elderly patients, as well as in treating some younger patients, where the prognosis does not warrant aggressive medical intervention and where the patients, if able to express their wishes, would probably refuse such treatment.

Physicians have learned a great deal from the new and emerging field of medical ethics about becoming aware of patients' preferences, which they elicit by encouraging the use of verbal or written "advance directives," or by holding discussions with family members who can report attitudes and values of the patient that might be relevant to making a decision to allow death to occur. Advance directives include legal instruments such as "living wills" and "durable powers of attorney for health care" (Kapp, 1989). They can also include conversations between the physician and the patient regarding the use or nonuse of life-sustaining treatments in the event of critical illness; in this case the patient's preferences are written down and become part of the medical record.

More and more physicians and hospitals are accepting the patient's right to die with dignity. More and more hospitals have explicit policies for do-not-resuscitate orders (Miles and Cranford, 1982). More and more physicians and hospitals are accepting the concept of hospice care for patients who are not likely to regain any meaningful level of existence. More and more state supreme courts, in cases of hopeless illness, have decided in favor of the patient's or the family's petition for the withdrawal of life-sustaining medical treatment (Wanzer et al., 1989).

There is still room for progress in this area, however, for many physicians and other personnel in hospitals and nursing homes are still unduly worried about their legal liability in such situations. They may continue to use medically unwarranted and morally unacceptable medical treatment because of their fear of legal repercussions if treatment is discontinued. Such fear is largely unwarranted, for there are few instances of successful lawsuits brought against physicians for withholding or withdrawing life-sustaining measures when the patient and the family have been involved in the decision, and when the treatment adheres to stated institutional protocols (Miles and Gomez, 1989).

Nonetheless, in the litigious environment of the United States the physician or the medical institution can never be entirely immune from lawsuits. Physicians need to reassert their moral courage to advocate the course of treatment most consistent with caring medical practice and respect for the patient's wishes. Malpractice reform and increasing attention to statutes that encourage the use of advance directives would enhance the physician's likelihood of making sensible decisions regarding the care of hopelessly ill patients. It is most important that such decisions should continue to be based on the individual case, not on some sweeping policy or regulation, especially not on a policy that uses age as the decisive criterion for withholding intensive medical treatment.

For example, some families would want the physician to administer antibiotics to treat pneumonia in a parent with advanced Alzheimer's disease, even though the quality of that parent's life may be very low when assessed by others. The family may find simple physical caregiving to be meaningful to both the aged parent and the caretakers, and may not regard it as too burdensome, even in the home setting. At the same time, treatments such as cardiopulmonary resuscitation or mechanical ventilation, which are ordinarily used only in comparatively severe life-threatening episodes, may not be indicated for the same patient because the burdens of treatment for that patient would not be justified by the chances of success. In most such instances, the situation is seen by everyone concerned as offering no chance of the patient's recovery, and no disagreement arises. In other instances, families and physicians together come to such decisions. The decision reached depends on the patient's condition, the views of the patient and the family, and their relationship with the physician.

Decisions to withhold medical treatment are never easy, nor should they be. Struggling through the management of such cases should help physicians to become more sensitive to the needs of hopelessly ill patients, to the subtleties of clinical treatment decisions for the most frail elderly patients, and to the skills needed for communication with families who are under the stress of caring for a severely impaired relative.

What Are the Basic Values of Medicine?

Concerns about health care expenditures have raised some fundamental questions about the goals of medicine. What is medical care for? Is it for prolonging the lives of the disabled, or is it only for prolonging the lives of those who can be functioning members of society? Is a person's functioning to be measured in terms of economic productivity, and is economic productivity the predominant value by which to judge human life? Should the criteria for medical treatment be different for patients who are financially covered by publicly funded programs such as Medicare and Medicaid than for patients who are privately insured and those who can pay out-of-pocket?

These issues arise not only in regard to elderly persons but also in regard to expenditures for the long-term care of disabled children and young adults. Such questions are now being raised increasingly often, especially with regard to intensive care for infants with severe birth defects. New developments in the care of AIDS patients, treatments that promise longer life expectancy but not complete recovery, will probably raise similar concerns.

In spite of these conflicting values—cost containment and patients' right to medical care—the basic values of medicine remain the same as before: the preservation of life, the relief of suffering, and respect for patients. Advances in medical technology have made the implementation of these values more complex, for in addition to problems of cost containment, the striving to save life often creates great emotional burdens for patients and families, and sometimes seems to conflict with a humanistic approach to patient care. The latter problem needs clarification if we are to understand the goals of modern medicine in an aging society.

It is useful to realize that policy controversies about the costs of medical care and about setting limits to medical interventions for old people center around two different models of medicine. Although these models are not necessarily mutually exclusive, and although, for some patients, the models may lead to identical modes of care, their primary goals are nevertheless clearly distinguishable.

The "Heroic" Model of Medicine

The overriding goal of the heroic model of medicine is the extension of life. In this model, life itself is of irreducible value; and the goal for the medical researcher, as well as for the practicing physician, is to postpone death, regardless of the patient's quality of life and regardless of the cost of treatment. In its most simplistic form, the heroic model of medicine does not ask whether a death is premature, appropriate, or acceptable, but asks only how death, the enemy, can be held at bay. The physician experiences the death of a patient as a personal failure, and perhaps also as an unwelcome reminder of his or her own mortality.

The intoxicating successes of medical technology—such as routine cardiac monitoring and defibrillation, mechanical ventilation, and kidney dialysis—that appeared during the 1960s probably created a receptive environment for the growth and acceptance of this heroic model. Certainly this model did not exist in earlier periods of history, when the physician's role was as much to "abide with" families during the illness of a patient as to dramatically rescue the patient from death.

Perceptions of the inhumanity of highly technical medical care, especially in cases of terminal disease, have led to public expressions of frustration with the heroic model of medicine, especially by those who demand a right to "die with dignity." Researchers in thanatology (the study of death and dying) have examined why some physicians are unable to accept their own mortality and why other physicians can deal patiently and compassionately with their patients' deaths. Accordingly, thanatologists have suggested a range of educational and institutional changes to enable society to deal better with death and dying. One result has been the development of hospice care for patients with terminal illness. Another is the increased discussion of death and dying in the medical curriculum.

The heroic model of medicine has brought with it, of course, an emphasis on medical research, as symbolized by the growth of the U.S. National Institutes of Health, by the "wars" on cancer and on heart disease, and by the enthusiastic search for "cures." In medical training, however, this model has resulted in much less emphasis being placed on the management of chronic disease and on the treatment of the more common but not life-threatening problems that patients present, and more emphasis being placed on the diagnosis and treatment of less common but potentially curable disorders.

The heroic model has indeed won many heroic victories, and it is a glamorous and exciting model both for health care professionals and for the public at large. It is undeniable that the goal of a longer life and the fantasy of being rescued from death are attractive to most people.

However, the heroic model cannot deal with uncertainty, with decline, or with death. It cannot encompass the wide range of clinical experience or the humility and compassion that are necessary for medical care in a society characterized by increasing longevity and increasing chronic illness.

The Humanistic Model of Medicine

In the second model of medicine, the one called the "humanistic" model, the primary goal is the improvement of the quality of life. In this model, the physician is much more likely to accept the patient on the patient's own terms and to establish goals of treatment which improve or maintain that person's level of functioning and quality of life. The prolongation of the patient's life is not necessarily what the physician strives for if that is not the patient's goal.

One example of this humanistic model is seen in the palliative approach of hospice care, in which the aim is to control the patient's symptoms and to make the patient comfortable. The application of this model is fairly straightforward in the care of a patient who is suffering from a clearly terminal illness and whose life expectancy is measured in days or weeks. However, in the great majority of elderly patients, multiple chronic diseases are the rule. The distinction between treatment aimed at improving the quality of life for these persons and treatment aimed at life prolongation is not so clear. This is particularly true in patients of advanced old age.

The humanistic approach must extend to psychological, social, and other issues, and it often requires a multidisciplinary team approach. This is especially true in treating older people, because the health problems that cause them distress often cannot be dealt with simply by prescriptions or surgery. The old patient may require economic, psychological, and social support, possibly including improved transportation, suitable housing, education about nutrition, and more.

In the humanistic model, the physician seeks medical interventions that place a low burden on the patient and have a high likelihood of benefit. The physician is unlikely to subject a patient to a procedure or treatment that involves a great deal of pain, as, for example, in resuscitating a frail elderly patient where there is only a small likelihood of improvement in that patient's life after the treatment ends.

In many of the interventions that improve the quality of life, particularly in a very old person, the prolongation of life may be an inevitable side effect. A good example is when a physician recently prescribed a pacemaker for a 99-year-old woman who was experiencing attacks of fainting caused by cardiac arrhythmia. While it may be agreed that extraordinary efforts to prolong the patient's life would be unseemly, "contraindicated," or perhaps even rejected by the patient herself, nonetheless the implantation of a pacemaker will prevent her from continually fainting, and thus falling and risking a broken hip, with its likelihood of protracted disability. The goal of such treatment is palliative—to prevent falling and potential fracture—but the salutary effect that the pacemaker will have on her heart rhythm will undoubtably extend her life.

The observation that treatments that improve life and those that extend life are often indistinguishable applies to almost any palliative measure, ranging from the administration of insulin to persons with diabetes and the administration of oxygen to persons who suffer from shortness of breath, to modern, technology-intensive treatments for heart failure or symptomatic malignancies.

A Model of Medicine for the Aging Society

Why is it that we are seeking a principle by which to limit medical treatment? Is it not obvious to the clinician when a certain treatment is or is not indicated? Clearly, physicians themselves often feel at sea, particularly in the care of very old patients. Old people are a new population to be served, and how best to serve them is a question that has only recently been receiving attention in medical research and training (Cassel, 1987). The guidelines are not clear, and they become especially problematic in a society in which physicians are pressured to be the gatekeepers of society's wealth and to prevent the wasteful use of dollars on people who will not "benefit."

Who is to decide what it means for the patient to benefit? Must the patient's life also be of present benefit to society? One assumption often made in this discourse is that if we could identify the best-functioning elderly person, or perhaps the best-functioning person of any age, we could then produce proper guidelines and would then know to whom medical care should best be offered.

Optimal Care Only for Those Who Function Well?

Various indexes of functioning have been explored by investigators who believe that when the patient's quality of life is very low, it is appropriate to limit medical care, particularly life-extending medical care. Those who are arguing for the rationing of medical care for old people advocate such decisions in treating all older patients, even those who are not extremely ill or terminally ill, and the establishment of a general policy of this kind.

This would mean that over time medical care would be provided more often to old persons whose quality of life is relatively high—those who are often described as "aging successfully"—than to persons whose quality of life is low.

One problem is that, for many observers, the quality of life is defined in reductionist terms, as the level of functioning. In one notable instance, it has been defined in even more reductionist terms, as the level of physiologic functioning; in that instance, old persons who score high on tests of half a dozen physiologic functions are termed the "successful agers" (Rowe and Kahn, 1987).

If the level of functioning were to become, for policy makers, the criterion for determining the type of medical care to be provided, the outcome would be to give more medical care to those who are physically and mentally able, and less to those who are disabled. Not only would such a policy increase inequities in the allocation of health care, but it also raises other underlying ethical questions. Except for the most extremely ill patients, about whom disagreements are rare, how and by whom shall the patient's quality of life be determined? At what point is any given type of medical care no longer warranted? Is it acceptable, on ethical grounds, to make such distinctions and then to act on them, in the interest of cost containment?

If such a policy mandating old-age-based rationing of medical care were to be implemented, it would represent a major departure from the prevailing goal of medicine in our society. Perhaps more importantly, however, for most persons in the society it would represent, on ethical grounds, too high a price for the society to pay.

Optimal Care for All Persons?

The goal of medicine our society has been pursuing to date is to provide medical care that enhances not only the level of functioning but also the quality of life for all persons. Today that goal focuses more sharply than before on the expectation that over time a larger and larger proportion of the population will age "successfully." However, to produce a population most of whose members are at high levels of functioning may not necessarily be the optimum, or even the preferred, goal for a society like our own.

We have been experiencing a tidal wave of improvement in health, which is most clearly shown by the dramatic rise in average life expectancy. Although not all subgroups in the population are experiencing the same rapid gains, still there is no disagreement that the population as a whole has benefited enormously. There is a price to be paid for this, however: the one implied by the metaphor "The rising tide lifts all boats equally." That is, the frail as well as the sturdy are being lifted. Although most people who survive to an advanced old age remain quite vigorous and independent, we shall never be without a certain number who, while they too are now surviving, do so with significant disability and with great need for both medical and social support.

In light of all the advantages of an increase in life expectancy, is the task of caring for those who are aging less than successfully too great a price for our society to pay? A related question is the one already suggested above: namely, whether our measures of success are too narrow. We have learned the sobering lessons of eugenics from a recent society in which only those persons who were regarded as the most highly functioning were allowed to survive. Equally sobering, in the present context, is the fact that the genocide practiced by the Nazis began with physician-supported "mercy killing" of persons who were retarded, mentally ill, or aged and infirm.

Whether or not our own society would move along the same downward path is debatable, but our medical successes have led some of us to view chronic disability and dependence, no matter what the cause, as simply undesirable, as a drain on our resources, or as our failure. These attitudes could lead to a harsh and unforgiving society, one that values only the healthy or only those who can pay their own way. It would be a regressive society, rather than one that reflects the successes of modern civilization. The civilized society allocates resources, both financial and emotional, for including in the life of the community those of its members who are less fortunate, and for providing care to them.

Embracing the Aging Society

Some observers believe that caring for disabled elderly persons will be an unbearable burden on society and will enervate and destroy us. Perhaps, to the contrary, society will benefit if it is challenged by the need to care for the vulnerable and the frail. Society's vitality and productivity may be improved if it learns how to sustain the lessons of compassion and how best to care for those who need care—in so doing, developing attributes such as loyalty and trust—as well as how to increase community cohesion.

Caring for the disabled may lead, also, to the creation of institutions of medicine and health care which reflect the needs of the modern society—to provide more home care and long-term care, and to be more prudent in the use of expensive medical commodities of unproven value (Brook and Lohr, 1986). We might learn to cut costs by using governmental power to limit the profits generated by entrepreneurial pharmaceutical and medical equipment companies, and to discourage their marketing practices that lead to wasteful overutilization of high-priced therapeutic and diagnostic procedures. We might learn instead how to create policies and methods for the strict assessment of technological procedures. Modern technology is not an evil in itself, but its indiscriminate use is medically inappropriate and wasteful, for it often diverts resources that could be used for long-term or preventive care (see Hiatt, 1987, especially pp. 13–33).

The appropriateness of any technology or treatment must be decided separately for each individual patient. The physician's role is to understand the potential efficacy or lack of efficacy of a given treatment, and to recommend treatment consistent with the patient's condition and the patient's values, regardless of the patient's age, sex, skin color, or income level.

Medicine in today's world needs to embrace the changing society in which people are living so much longer, and to create a humane model of medical care that fits the new social realities. It should focus not on setting age limits for medical care but, rather, on adding opportunities for a continuing sense of the value of life, especially for the very old. In this approach one is neither nihilistic nor fatalistic about the chances of helping old as well as young people.

The complexity of modern medicine requires an integration of the heroic and the humanistic, the technologic and the psychosocial approaches to health. The welfare of the individual patient is the measure by which any medical intervention must be assessed. The aging of our society, and the critique of modern medicine it has engendered, can lead to a medical practice that is better for all patients, and therefore for the society at large. At the same time, it requires a careful examination of the complexities involved. Otherwise it could lead to discrimination against sick and disabled persons and to the dehumanization of our society.

References

Brody, J.A., and Schneider, E.L. (1983). Aging, natural death, and the compression of morbidity: another view. *New England Journal of Medicine, 309,* 854–856.

Brook, R.H., and Lohr, K.N. (1986). Will we need to ration effective health care? *Issues in Science and Technology, 3*(1), 68–77.

Callahan, D. (1987). *Setting limits: medical goals in an aging society.* New York: Simon & Schuster.

Callahan, D. (1990). *What kind of life: the limits of medical progress.* New York: Simon & Schuster.

Campbell, A., Converse, P., and Rodgers, W. (1976). *The quality of American life.* New York: Russell Sage Foundation.

Carlson, R.J. (1975). *The end of medicine.* New York: John Wiley & Sons.

Cassel, C.K. (1987). Certification: another step for geriatric medicine. *Journal of the American Medical Association, 258,* 1518–1519.

Daniels, N. (1988). *Am I my parents' keeper? an essay on justice between the young and the old.* New York: Oxford University Press.

Fries, J.F. (1980). Aging, natural death, and the compression of morbidity. *New England Journal of Medicine, 303,* 130–135.

Harris, L., and Associates (1975). *The myth and reality of aging in America.* Washington, D.C.: National Council on the Aging.

Harris, L., and Associates (1981). *Aging in the eighties.* Washington, D.C.: National Council on the Aging.

Hiatt, H.H. (1987). *America's health in the balance.* New York: Harper & Row.

Hing, E. (1987). *Use of nursing homes by the elderly: preliminary data from the 1985 National Nursing Home Survey, Advance Data No. 135.* Hyattsville, Md: National Center for Health Statistics, May 14.

Illich, I. (1976). *Medical nemesis: the expropriation of health.* New York: Pantheon Books.

Kane, R.L., and Kane, R.A. (1990). Health care for older people: organizational and policy issues. In R.H. Binstock and L.K. George, eds, *Handbook of aging and the social sciences* (3rd ed.), pp. 415–437. San Diego: Academic Press.

Kapp, M. (1989). Medical treatments and the physician's legal duties. In C.K. Cassel and D. Reisenberg, eds., *Geriatric medicine* (2nd ed.), pp. 623–639. New York: Springer-Verlag.

Katz, S., Branch, L.G., Branson, M.H., Papsidero, J.A., Beck, J.C., and Greer, D.S. (1983). Active life expectancy. *New England Journal of Medicine, 309,* 1218–1224.

Knowles, J.H., ed. (1977). Doing better and feeling worse: health in the United States. *Daedalus: Journal of the American Academy of Arts and Sciences, 106*(1).

Lamm, R.D. (1987). Ethical health care for the elderly: are we cheating our children? In T.M. Smeeding, ed., *Should medical care be rationed by age?,* pp. xi–xv. Totowa, N.J.: Rowman & Littlefield.

Lubitz, J., and Prihoda, R. (1984). The uses and costs of Medicare services in the last two years of life. *Health Care Financing Review, 5*(3), 117–131.

Maddox, G. (1986). Dynamics of population aging: a changing, changeable profile. In *America's aging workforce: a Traveler's symposium,* pp. 30–37. Hartford, Conn.: Traveler's Insurance Co.

Manton, K.G. (1990). Mortality and morbidity. In R.H. Binstock and L.K. George, eds., *Handbook of aging and the social sciences* (3rd ed.), pp. 64–90. San Diego: Academic Press.

Miles, S.H., and Cranford, R. (1982). The do-not-resuscitate order in a teaching hospital. *Annals of Internal Medicine, 96,* 660–664.

Miles, S.H., and Gomez, C.F. (1989). *Protocols for elective use of life-sustaining treatments.* New York: Springer Publishing Co.

Olshansky, S.J., and Ault, B.A. (1986). The fourth stage of the epidemiologic transition: the age of delayed degenerative diseases. *Milbank Memorial Fund Quarterly/Health and Society, 64,* 355–391.

Rowe, J.W., and Kahn, R.L. (1987). Human aging: usual and successful. *Science, 237,* 143–149.

Schneider, E.L. (1989). Options to control the rising health care costs of older Americans. *Journal of the American Medical Association, 261,* 907.

Scitovsky, A.A. (1984). The high cost of dying: what do the data show? *Milbank Memorial Fund Quarterly/Health and Society, 62,* 591–608.

Shock, N.W., Greulich, R., Andres, R., Arenberg, D., Costa, P., Jr., Lakatta, E., and Tobin, J. (1984). *Normal human aging: the Baltimore longitudinal study of aging.* Washington, D.C.: U.S. Government Printing Office.

U.S. Bureau of the Census, Office of the Actuary (1988). *The centenarians.* Washington, D.C.: U.S. Government Printing Office.

U.S. Senate, Special Committee on Aging, in conjunction with the American Association of Retired Persons, the Federal Council on the Aging, and the U.S. Administration on Aging (1987). *Aging America: trends and projections.* Washington, D.C.: U.S. Government Printing Office.

Waitzkin, H. (1983). *The second sickness: contradictions of capitalist health care.* New York: Free Press.

Wanzer, S., Federman, D., Adelstein, S.J., Cassel, C., Cassem, E., Cranford, R., Hook, E., Lo, B., Mortel, C., Safar, P., Stone, A., and van Eys, J. (1989). The physician's responsibility toward hopelessly ill patients: a second look. *New England Journal of Medicine, 320,* 844–849.

5

Age-based Rationing and the Law: An Exploration

NANCY NEVELOFF DUBLER, L.L.B., and
CHARLES P. SABATINO, J.B.

The United States is a litigious society. It is natural for Americans to resolve in court many disputes that, in other societies, are often resolved by a combination of administrative decisions and informal negotiation. This litigiousness leads to a deluge of civil and tort suits designed to adjudicate alleged wrongs and provide monetary remedies for loss. It also results in constitutional litigation that not only judges individual rights but, in so doing, provides broad moral and legal principles by which individuals' actions will be measured.

The official implementation of one or more of the contemporary proposals that life-sustaining health care be categorically denied to older persons would inevitably seed a myriad of individual suits seeking to maximize available medical services. The notion of public rationing of health care for elderly persons also conjures up a host of constitutional challenges that would dissect the legal and ethical underpinnings of society's decisions and ultimately determine whether age-based rationing would survive the scrutiny of federal courts applying previously established principles of equity and legislative power.

In this chapter we will examine a number of areas of developed or evolving law which could prove important in these hypothetical constitutional challenges. We will offer some initial comments on the general legal status of elderly persons in the United States: in the common law (with special reference to guardianship law); in modern social policy as expressed in federal legislation; and in constitutional law.

Turning specifically to health care, we will briefly consider the present condition of the asserted "right" to health care and the question of whether elderly persons have a right to life-sustaining care. In this context we will consider whether cases addressing both issues of terminal care and abortion might have some bearing on the future resolution of these issues. Next we will discuss potential constitutional and legislative barriers to proposals that attempt to exclude elderly people from participation in certain health care benefits. Finally, we will examine some of the present systems of formal and informal health care rationing, brought about largely by interlocking federal legislation, regulatory interpretation, and rule making, and consider how far this informal rationing could be extended into a coherent national policy of rationing health care for all older Americans.

One caveat before we begin: Predicting the outcome of constitutional litigation is the modern equivalent of soothsaying or reading a crystal ball—and it is probably only half as effective. The Supreme Court is notorious for the independently evolving legal philosophies of its members. The terms liberal and conservative, often applied to individual justices, hardly suffice to describe the complex personal decisions—let alone the collective decisions—reached by the Court. Moreover, the aggregate character of the Supreme Court and its analytical proclivities change over time, sometimes at geologic rates, sometimes with jumps and jitters. A search for legal guideposts needs to reach beyond present politics and personalities.

Despite these confounding realities, we will suggest some of the elements that will certainly be found in future legal challenges concerning age-based rationing, and speculate on their relative value. While we have neither the prescience nor the temerity to pronounce on the eventual outcomes, we will conclude that the law's vision (both judicial and statutory) of elderly persons has evolved over time in a way that suggests that its reception of the notion of age-based rationing of health care would be reluctant, although not outright hostile to the proposition. Indeed, under a rigorous and narrow interpretation of constitutional cases, such rationing, at least from the judicial perspective, might be acceptable.

Elderly People: Position in Law

The Common Law and the Evolution of Guardianship

There is now something legally special about being old, but this was not always the case. Until the middle of the last century, when England began experimenting with prototype reform and welfare legislation, elderly persons were largely dependent on the care and protection of family members. Some of the most visible and destitute would end their days in the almshouses that most communities maintained.

Since the mid-fifteenth century, with the passage in England of the law *De Praerogativa Regis*, there had been the concept of special protection for those lacking the ability to care for themselves. This law, which permitted the king to manage the lands and profits of estates, was basically for "idiots,"that is, those born without the capacity for reason, and "lunatics," those who later in life lost that capacity (Brakel, 1985, p. 10) As the original model for present-day guardianship and conservatorship statutes, it might have promised supervision and support at least for demented elder persons but for one fact—it was only applicable to the propertied class, where chaos in the management of the affairs of the wealthy might contribute to disorder in the realm.

Following this pattern, several of the American colonies passed legislation designed to protect the estates of "insane persons" (Deutsch, 1949). Gradually, this basic schema of legally sanctioned paternalism received a clear statutory foundation in all states in the form of guardianship laws. These laws, however, shared the flaws of the original conception in that they were largely focused on the management of property and not on the care of the elderly (*In re Fisher*, 1989; Schmidt et al., 1981, pp. 10–14; Spring and Dubler, 1990). Guardianship law has undergone a slow but significant evolution over the last 20 years. The major themes revealed by an analysis of that evolution provide an instructive perspective from which to view some of the U.S. legal system's guiding assumptions about the aged and the process of aging.

The first theme concerns the refinement of the legal concept of "incompetency," the historically amorphous legal prerequisite for guardianship. The legal standards for incompetency originally relied on "status-" or diagnosis-based tests, under which old age itself is virtually presumed to be a disability. Status-based tests require that the individual be suffering from some kind of diagnosable condition and that, as a result of the condition, he or she be unable to properly manage his or her property or person. The lists of disabling conditions recited in state laws have commonly included mental illness, mental deficiency, physical illness, drug addiction, and advanced age itself. Indeed, a 1986 survey showed that some 35 states listed "advanced age," "old age," or "senility" as a statutory ground for declaring incompetency or incapacity (American Bar Association, 1986; Frosberg, 1986). The bias obvious in these statutes is that age itself is a disabling condition.

Since the early 1970s, a growing number of states have moved away from the status-based test toward a functional test, influenced strongly by modern clinical notions of incapacity, which were developed to determine whether a person has the ability to provide informed consent to medical treatment. A functional test essentially examines an individual's ability to understand key information, cognitively process that information, and communicate a choice (Parry, 1985). A purely functional test eschews general presumptions about aged persons and attempts to focus objectively on the particular abilities and circumstances of the individual.

Guardianship reform has accelerated noticeably since 1987, when the Associated Press (1987) published the results of an extensive national investigation it had conducted exposing widespread problems with state guardianship systems. A number of states have begun to revamp their procedures and modify their definitions of incapacity, and the changes have included the repeal of "advanced age" as a criterion for incapacity. The American Bar Association itself has consistently advocated the elimination of age as a consideration in determining incompetency (American Bar Association, 1987; American Bar Association, 1989b).

A second significant theme is really a corollary of the functional approach to capacity; it can be described as a growing appreciation of the "situation-specific" nature of an individual's capacity. On one level, jurisprudence has always recognized differing standards of capacity for differing transactions, such as making a will, marrying, entering a contract, driving a car, standing trial, or managing one's property and personal affairs. However, a finding of incapacity in this last category was historically the most global, justifying the most intrusive curtailments of personal liberty. Under the old order, a finding of incompetency automatically abrogated the full spectrum of the ward's civil rights, including the rights to vote, to marry, and to contract (Parry, 1985). This blunt, all-or-nothing approach has given way to a more finely tuned recognition of individual functional capacities: that is, courts are now expected to better differentiate the individual abilities of allegedly incompetent persons, and the authority of a guardian is limited to only those specific areas of deficiency articulated in the judicial order. Concepts of limited, partial, and temporary guardianship exemplify this trend.

The third theme concerns the growing recognition of the importance of procedural due process in the context of guardianship. Procedural protections work to ensure that decisions are made fairly and with full appreciation of the individual's needs and interests. Much of the statutory reform regarding guardianship in recent years has focused on strengthening these protections, ensuring for instance, that the putative ward has the right to notice of the proceedings, representation by an attorney, an impartial expert evaluation, attendance at all judicial proceedings, and cross-examination of witnesses (American Bar Association, 1989a). It is noteworthy that even before the era of guardianship reform, the law recognized a presumption of competency (at least for white male landowners); in establishing incompetency, the burden of proof was placed on the shoulders of the petitioning party.

This rise of procedural due process reflects the same type of evolution that was seen a decade earlier in the field of involuntary civil commitment. Perhaps the lag in the field of guardianship is attributable to a more deeply entrenched assumption of benefit paternalism in this area, coupled with the fact that the human consequences are less visible. Guardianship lacks the asylum imagery so easily associated with civil commitment.

Taken together, these trends suggest an ongoing refinement of the law's response to individual needs, abilities, and interests, especially with respect to the elderly individuals who make up the majority of the allegedly disabled persons who come under the scrutiny of the legal system. In summary,

> Just as in many instances modern brain surgeons have discarded the scalpel in favor of the laser beam, courts and legislators need to replace outmoded legal concepts that were once useful for making determinations about mentally disabled people with new concepts that are designed to examine individual needs and individual rights. (Parry, 1985, p. 379).

The waning of misguided age assumptions and the fine-tuning of the law's response to disabled persons in the area of guardianship law suggests an analytic evolution increasingly intolerant of policies that could deprive aged persons of rights and benefits merely on the basis of their status as elderly. However, guardianship law and the common law generally do not determine the course of national health policy. They are instructive and predictive to the extent that their intellectual themes are relevant to other areas of law and policy. The legislative and constitutional discussions below will reveal some analogous analytic themes in these other areas as well.

Federal Legislation

The most visible forum of activity defining the legal position of elderly people in American society has been the United States Congress. The passage of the Social Security Act in 1935, several housing assistance enactments since the Housing Act of 1937, the creation of Medicare and Medicaid in 1965, the Older Americans Act of 1965, the Age Discrimination in Employment Act (ADEA) of 1967, the Employee Retirement Income Security Act (ERISA) of 1974, the Age Discrimination Act (ADA) of 1975, and subsequent amendments to these and other federal statutes have provided a complicated array of age-based and need-based entitlements and rights that reflect two opposing poles of social policy makers' perceptions about the elderly.

On the one hand, elderly persons are perceived as vulnerable, dependent, and in need, a view that parallels some of the traditional assumptions about the elderly in the common law. Under this premise, the history of federal legislation has shown a fairly consistent expansion of benefits for older Americans.

On the other hand, enactments such as the ADEA represent deliberate federal attempts to counteract social stereotypes of elderly persons as frail and incapable. The stated purpose of the ADEA is

> to promote employment of older persons based on their ability rather than age; to prohibit arbitrary age discrimination in employment; to help employers and workers find ways of meeting problems arising from the impact of age on employment. (Age Discrimination in Employment Act, 1967, sec. 621[6])

This latter view can be seen as a parallel to that evident in modern guardianship reform. Both stand on a premise that an elderly citizen is entitled to be a full participant in all the rights and privileges of society unless it can be proven that this should not be the case. Where an individual's incapacities preclude full participation, those incapacities are to be narrowly construed based upon relevant facts and not upon age.

The two poles certainly suggest a conflict in assumptions, but it is arguable that the conflict operates more as a creative tension in social policy than as a contradiction. Thus, we could describe it as a process of lowering the threshold for full and active participation in society, while increasing the benefits available to those who fall below that threshold. As we shall see below, this policy tension has specific relevance to the issue of the age-based rationing of health care.

Constitutional Law

Distinctions based on group classifications are common in most legislation. In general, statutes either impose responsibilities on—or grant or deny benefits to—groups, whether they be taxpayers, parents, sport fishermen, pickle producers, or elderly people. When these distinctions are challenged on constitutional grounds, they are invariably measured against equal protection requirements. The Fourteenth Amendment provides that "no State shall . . . deny to any person within its jurisdiction the equal protection of the laws." While this clause is not applicable to the federal government, it has been held that most acts by the federal government that would deny equal protection constitute a "deprivation of liberty" within the Fifth Amendment's due process clause (*Bolling v. Sharpe*, 1954).

The "rational basis" test. The usual test for determining whether a classification is permissible under equal protection analysis is the rational basis test. This test requires only that the classification be "rationally related" to a proper state interest. Under this test, a challenged statute must be accorded a presumption of constitutionality if any set of facts may reasonably be thought of to justify it (Rotunda et al., 1986). It is highly deferential to legislative discretion, and consequently, the Supreme Court rarely finds a violation of equal protection under this low-level test.

The "strict scrutiny" test. The courts utilize a much more stringent test, referred to as the "strict scrutiny" test, if a legislative classification seems to interfere with "the exercise of a fundamental right or operates to the peculiar disadvantage of a suspect class" (*Massachusetts Board of Retirement v. Murgia* [hereafter *Murgia*, 1976], p. 2566). Under this test, a classification will be held to violate equal protection unless found to be necessary to promote a compelling state interest. Challenges to legislative classifications have a relatively high likelihood of success under this strict scrutiny test.

The "suspect class" test. In recent constitutional litigation, the Supreme Court has only once considered whether there was something special about being old that would qualify the elderly as a suspect class for equal protection purposes. In the case of *Murgia* (1976), the court found that elder persons—or more specifically, state policemen over the age of 50—did not constitute a suspect class for purposes of equal protection analysis.

Lieutenant Colonel Robert D. Murgia was retired from the Uniformed Branch of the Massachusetts State Police pursuant to a Massachusetts statute that required state police officers with 20 years of service to be retired upon reaching the age of 50. Officer Murgia, who was in excellent health and fully capable of performing the tasks of an officer, challenged this rule on equal protection grounds. The Supreme Court rejected this claim and upheld the law. It stated:

> The primary function of the Uniformed Branch of the Massachusetts State Police is to protect persons and property and maintain law and order . . . there is a general relationship between advancing age and decreasing physical ability to respond to the demands of the job . . . The testimony clearly established that the risk of physical failure, particularly in the cardiovascular system, increases with age, and that the number of individuals in a given age group incapable of performing stress functions increases with the age of the group. (*Murgia*, 1976, pp. 2565–2566)

Further on in its opinion, the Court defined a suspect class as one

saddled with such disabilities, or subjected to such a history of purposeful unequal treatment, or relegated to such a position of political powerlessness as to command extraordinary protection from the majoritarian political process. While treatment of the aged in this Nation has not been wholly free of discrimination, such persons, unlike, say, those who have been discriminated against on the basis of race or national origin, have not experienced a history of purposeful unequal treatment or been subjected to unique disabilities on the basis of stereotyped characteristics not truly indicative of their abilities. (*Murgia*, 1976, p. 2567)

Thus, on its face, the constitutional status of elderly Americans appears to be no different than that of any group of citizens. Special consideration is not constitutionally mandated. However, below we will address some factors that could justify a different outcome for older persons who are fighting not for continued employment but instead for continuation of their lives.

Is There a Right to "Life-sustaining" Health Care?

In the United States there is a right to health care if a patient can reach a provider and pay for the care. This somewhat cynical characterization of the practical limitations of securing health care reflects the fact that no generally or universally applicable legal right to health care exists in this country. By now, a general constitutional right to health care seems to be beyond discussion. No serious scholar could assert that either the explicit language of the Constitution or the philosophical identification of "fundamental" rights creates an enforceable constitutional right to care.

Such a right has been recognized only in circumstances involving incarceration or commitment. For example, inmates in prisons and jails have a constitutional right to health care under interpretations of the Eighth Amendment. The court has reasoned that to put someone in prison where he or she cannot secure care, and subsequently not to provide care, can result in precisely the sort of "cruel and unusual" pain and suffering which the Eighth Amendment was designed to prohibit. Inmates therefore have a right to care, and correctional officials have a duty to provide care that does not manifest a "deliberate indifference to the serious medical needs" of inmates (*Estelle v. Gamble*, 1976; p. 292).

Similarly, mentally retarded persons who are involuntarily committed possess a constitutional right to liberty, which includes rights to adequate food, shelter, clothing, and medical care (*Youngberg v. Ro-*

mero, 1982). Although the Supreme Court has refrained from explicitly recognizing a general right to treatment for all institutionalized persons, numerous lower courts and the majority of state legislatures have formalized this basic entitlement (Weiner, 1985).

"The Right to Die"

Despite the lack of a general, legally enforceable right to health care in the United States, there may be some notion of a "right to life-sustaining care," based, ironically, on the collected body of cases that have established the right to refuse life-sustaining treatment, more popularly referred to as the "right to die." It is sometimes quipped these days that, because of its approach to abortion policy and the lack of health care for children, the federal government is interested in children "from conception to birth." So too, the federal government may be interested in elderly persons "from sickness to death," but only if life itself is imperiled.

One caution is required here. Any putative right to life-sustaining care will itself beg the question of how far such a right can be limited by the scarcity or the costliness of resources. Moreover, even though a right to life-sustaining care may be a potential shield against age-based rationing at the end of life, it is fraught with dangers, as we will see, for general "access-to-care" policies and for the right to refuse care.

Since the case of Karen Ann Quinlan (*In re Quinlan*, 1976 [hereafter *Quinlan*, 1976]) courts have struggled to fashion rules that support the rights and the autonomy of patients while they protect the larger interest of society. In one of the earlier cases (*Superintendent of Belchertown State School v. Saikewicz*, 1978 [hereafter *Saikewicz*, 1978]), the Massachusetts Supreme Judicial Court identified four interests of the state as a party in litigation about the termination of care: protecting life, preventing suicide, protecting innocent third parties, and protecting the integrity of the medical profession.

Most right-to-die cases today involve choices about terminating life-sustaining care for a patient incapable of making a decision, when such termination will result in the death of the patient. The claim is generally made that the patient provided guidance, when capable of choosing, to indicate that he or she would want care withdrawn (*In re Eichner*, 1981; *In re Storer*, 1981; *In re Westchester Country Medical Center ex rel. O'Connor*, 1988 [hereafter *O'Connor*, 1988]). Sometimes the evidence of past choice is unclear and a court will permit the present care decision to be made on a basis of "substituted judgment," that is, in answer to the question "What would this patient tell us if he or she could communicate?" To answer this question requires extrapolation from the patient's past pattern of life and demonstrated behaviors.

Finally, some decisions are made without reference to explicit or inferred personal choice, even when the decision itself claims otherwise; rather, they are made on the basis of a "best interest" principle. Such cases are the most troubling, as they require implementing the judgments of others to determine care for the patient (e.g. *Saikewicz*, 1978).

The decisions in these cases, many of which involved elderly patients, have varied with respect to the substantive rules crafted and the procedures imposed. However, they have uniformly agreed that the termination of life support for patients is fraught with legal and moral uncertainty. Moreover, most scholars, as well as the courts that have addressed the issue, agree that there is no meaningful distinction between withdrawing and withholding care. Nonetheless, many cases, and the overwhelming majority of caregivers, behave as if a real and supportable distinction exists. This notion survives despite the argument that responsible medical practitioners should attempt an intervention to see if the patient will benefit, and if he or she does not, they may ethically discontinue the care. Somehow, the moral and medical framework appears to shift when the intervention is a sophisticated machine rather than an antibiotic.

The decisions in right-to-die cases may be taken to uphold the proposition that there is some right to the continuance of life-sustaining care unless there is guidance, in word or in behavior, from the patient's past to permit the discontinuance of care. These right-to-die cases have heavily focused the law on the extent of the state's interest in maintaining life, sometimes with rather odd implications. For example, under these cases, given the meager home care benefit under Medicare, the chronically ill, homebound elderly patient may have no access to adequate home care. However, that same person, after a stroke, in deep coma and on a ventilator, may have the right to have that care continued. Indeed, in some states, family members will be prevented from ordering the discontinuance of care (*Cruzan v. Director, Missouri Department of Health*, 1990; *O'Connor*, 1988).

The U.S. Supreme Court's decision in the case of Nancy Cruzan (*Cruzan*, 1990)—its first foray into the right to die—grants to the states considerable constitutional leeway to fashion decision-making standards and procedures as each state sees fit. While finding that a competent person has a constitutionally protected liberty interest in refusing unwanted medical treatment, the court held that the Constitution does not forbid states from establishing stringent standards of clear and convincing evidence for determining the wishes of incompetent persons. In those states with such standards, unless the patient has previously and expressly refused care, the "right to life-sustaining care" could become an obligation to accept care under any and all circumstances in which organ function can be artificially maintained—an ironic outcome. (For additional discussion of the *Cruzan* case, see chapter 7.)

These right-to-die/right-to-life cases are interesting in another way. They are fast becoming part of the agenda of the right-to-life lobbying groups. Increasing numbers of state legislatures, for example, have found their efforts to draft living-will legislation complicated by this lobby, which is gradually shifting its focus from abortion and neonatal decision making to decisions about terminal care of the elderly. In some 19 states with living-will legislation, the statutes include provisions that explicitly or implicitly restrict the extent to which a person can use an advance directive, or living will, to refuse artificial nutrition and hydration (Society for the Right to Die, 1988).

"The Right to Life"

The concept of a "right to life," first popularized in the abortion debate, may indeed have some relevance to elderly Americans. In the recently decided *Webster* case, the Supreme Court upheld certain restrictions on abortion passed by the Missouri legislature. In discussing the restrictions, the Court stated clearly that the provisions are constitutional as they further the "state's interest in protecting potential human life" (*Webster v. Missouri*, 1989, p. 3057). If the state has an interest in protecting the fetus, which is only a potential human life, one might wonder how much more weighty could or should be its interest in protecting the elderly near the end of their lives. Is the right to life the sort of fundamental right that an equal protection analysis will protect? Could discrimination against elderly persons in health care be prohibited by extending *Webster* and creating a new fundamental, and thus protectable, interest?

Unfortunately, even if the answer is yes, it may do little to prevent the rationing of health care for elderly citizens. The Supreme Court has been quite clear on this point since *Harris v. McRae*, in which it said:

> Regardless of whether the freedom of a woman to choose to terminate her pregnancy for health reasons lies at the core or the periphery of the due process liberty recognized in *Wade* [*Roe v. Wade*, the original abortion decision], it simply does not follow that a woman's freedom of choice carries with it a constitutional entitlement to the financial resources to avail herself of the full range of protected choices. (1980, p. 2688)

The Court reaffirmed this proposition in *Webster* when it stated that the Due Process Clauses generally confer no affirmative right to government aid, even where such aid may be necessary to secure life, liberty or property interests of which the government may not deprive the individual. (1989, p. 3051)

Thus, even if elderly people were relabeled a suspect class or were clearly protected by a fundamental right to life, that would not necessarily entitle them to the financial aid from Medicare or Medicaid needed to obtain that care.

There is one final avenue to explore in this brief discussion of possibly enforceable theories of rights. This avenue shifts the focus from the U.S. Constitution to federal statute, specifically to section 504 of the Rehabilitation Act of 1973. The act provides in part that

no otherwise qualified handicapped individual . . . shall, solely by reasons of his handicap, be excluded from the participation in, be denied the benefit of, or be subjected to discrimination under any program or activity receiving Federal financial assistance.

This section was used as one statutory basis for a series of lawsuits attempting, unsuccessfully, to establish the right of neonates to life-sustaining care, and, more importantly, the obligation of all health care providers to render that care. The intended impact of these suits was to restrict, if not destroy, the ability of parents and physicians to permit the death of multiply handicapped, imperiled newborns whose conditions are largely incompatible with life.

As a general proposition, it seems clear under interpretations of this statute that states may not discriminate against the handicapped in federally funded programs. It is less clear, but arguable, that where a state chooses to provide a service that is not required by Congress, but provides the service in a discriminatory manner, this section might still apply as an avenue of relief. The cases interpreting the clause make it clear that handicapped and disabled persons are entitled to treatment equal to that given to those without a handicap (Destro, 1986, p. 85). Could old age itself be a handicap? What about disabled elderly persons? Could we have the truly ridiculous result that healthy elderly persons could be denied benefits that their disabled age-mates would be required to receive? Needless to say, a program that rationed health care for elderly persons would try to avoid the pitfalls of section 504 of the Rehabilitation Act; or more likely, if Congress were to impose rationing through legislation, it would simultaneously amend section 504 to avoid conflict.

In summary, the legal routes by which elderly persons' access to life-sustaining care might be protected in the face of rationing are by no means certain to succeed. Even if such care is a fundamental right, the public funds necessary to ensure support for life may be withheld as a matter of law and public policy. Under the present federal schema, some protection might be provided by section 504 of the Rehabilitation Act; but any reasonable congressional rationing plan would also be likely to provide the necessary exclusion or exemption as part of its enabling package. Finally, any approach that ensures life-sustaining care, in contrast to health care generally, might be forced to rely on right-to-life cases and language. This is a course that could result in winning the battle against age-based rationing of certain treatments, but losing the war against curtailments of individual choice.

Can There Be Laws and Rules that Exclude Elderly Persons from Participation in Certain Benefits?

Benefits and Equal Protection

Most public benefit legislation necessarily denies certain benefits to some groups by virtue of the fact that the beneficiaries under any legislation must have some definitional limit. Earlier we described one avenue of equal protection analysis based on whether the group discriminated against is a suspect class. In *Murgia*, the Supreme Court found that the elderly did not constitute a suspect class. *Murgia* also considered the other potential trigger for applying a strict level of scrutiny, that is, whether a *fundamental right* was in question;

> Equal protection analysis requires strict scrutiny of a legislative classification only when the classification impermissibly interferes with the exercise of a fundamental right or operates to the peculiar disadvantage of a suspect class. (1976, p. 2566)

Fundamental rights and equal protection. The court listed the following fundamental rights: rights of a uniquely private nature (which have been connoted by the label "the right to privacy"), the right to vote, the right of interstate travel, the right to procreate, and the rights guaranteed by the First Amendment (*Murgia*, 1976, p. 2566, n. 3). Later commentators (Rotunda et al., 1986) omit the right to procreate and add two rights which they concede have never been the subject of a specific decision, but which they divine from a reading of cases in this area. They note first, a "right to fairness in the criminal process," and second, the "right to fairness in procedures concerning individual claims against governmental deprivations of life, liberty or property" (p. 85). It is this last right which we will examine here and which may ultimately prove most relevant and promising for this inquiry into legal barriers against age-based rationing of health care. If a "right to fairness" were to exist in situations involving the deprivation of life, could that be the basis for contesting certain rationing schemes? Is it realistic to posit that the Supreme Court might go in this direction?

In *Murgia*, the Court held that for purposes of equal protection analysis the right of governmental employment per se is not "fundamental," and the creation of a class of state police officers over 50 is not "suspect" (1976, p. 2567). Because of this finding, the rational basis test of constitutional suitability (which presumes validity) rather than the more stringent standard of strict scrutiny was used to measure the appropriateness of the state's law or regulation. Under this less rigorous review, the state "does not violate the Equal Protection Clause merely because the classifications made by its laws are imperfect" (*Murgia*, 1976, p. 2568; citing *Dandridge v. Williams*, 1970). For these reasons the Court upheld the Massachusetts rule.

Justice Marshall, dissenting in this case and other equal protection cases, and various other legal scholars have asserted that a rigid two-tiered analysis for equal protection purposes—one that upholds state action unless a fundamental right is implicated or unless the legislation is wholly unrelated to its objective—is too rigid for equitable and just adjudication. (Kirshenbaum, 1977, p. 771; *Murgia*, 1976, p. 2569). This is especially true because the Court seems reluctant to find additional fundamental rights (or suspect classes). In 1973, for example, it rejected education as a fundamental right (*San Antonio School District v. Rodriguez*, 1973), and declined to treat women as a suspect class (*Frontiero v. Richardson*, 1973, cited in *Murgia*, 1976, p. 2569).

A "sliding-scale" approach. As an alternative, Justice Marshall suggested a "sliding scale" approach, in which the degree of care with which a court scrutinizes a government program depends on the constitutional and societal importance of the interest adversely affected and the invidiousness of the basis upon which the classification is drawn (Kirshenbaum, 1977, p. 772). Given the extreme deference to state legislative behavior exhibited by the Supreme Court in recent terms, however, it seems unlikely that the present Court will either expand the categories of fundamental rights or define new suspect classes; nor is it likely to expressly develop a level of scrutiny intermediate between the low-level rational basis test and the more rigorous strict scrutiny test. This present Supreme Court seems exquisitely aware that

> the drawing of lines that create distinctions is peculiarly a legislative task and an unavoidable one. Perfection in making the necessary classifications

is neither possible nor necessary . . . such action by a legislature is presumed valid. (*Murgia*, 1976, p. 2567)

"Minimal scrutiny with a bite." In at least a few cases, however, some scholars interpret the Court to be applying a slightly more rigorous rational basis test, at least for gender discrimination cases—a test that has been labeled "minimal scrutiny with a bite." Under this test, the Court appears to require a "fair and substantial relationship between the means chosen to effectuate the legislative purpose and the objective itself" (Evans, 1977, p. 378). Despite this scholarly optimism in advancing protections for population subgroups, the Court has refused to refer to or to implement this test in most recent cases.

On the contrary, this present Supreme Court may be reinforcing a line of cases in which "extreme deference" is given to legislative action. These cases are alarming because in them the validity of the statute's purpose is never really considered. These cases suggest "that legislation will be accepted as valid if any reason is or can be advanced to support the challenged classification" (Evans, 1977, p. 382).

Benefits and Statutory Prohibitions against Age Discrimination

The Age Discrimination Act. The statute most explicitly relevant, to assuring that elderly persons are not excluded from participation in federal programs, yet least utilized for that purpose, is the Age Discrimination Act. The ADA provides that

> no person in the United States shall, on the basis of age be excluded from participation in, be denied the benefits of, or be subjected to discrimination under, any program or activity receiving federal financial assistance. (Age Discrimination Act, 1975, sec. 6102)

Would the ADA prevent the rationing of health care for elderly persons through federal policy? Despite the apparent meaning in this section, it is clear from the legislative debate and from other sections of the act that the purpose of the ADA was not to prohibit age discrimination, but only to prohibit that which is "unreasonable" (Silver, 1988, p. 1021). Moreover, it was not clear which sorts of discrimination Congress was trying to prohibit, although it was relatively clear that Congress "wished to prevent the establishment of maximum age limits for participation in federally assisted programs when those limits were based upon an assessment of the 'social worth' of older individuals" (p. 1030). However, the ADA exempts specific laws that use age as a criterion, and therefore, "if any age distinction is struck down, it can be validated by the passage of federal, state, or local legislation. If a legislative body makes a policy choice to permit an age distinction in a given program, the ADA will not be a barrier" (p. 1035). Although this makes discrimination in public policy theoretically possible, such discrimination must of course be politically feasible in order to happen.

Despite the relative weakness of the ADA when confronted with statutory bases for discrimination, it could be quite effective as a deterrent for local administrative or regulatory discrimination. It is designed to "prevent the use of age as a measure of qualification when other means of making that determination are available," although an individualized evaluation of elderly persons is only required if "it is feasible and will not undermine the program" (Silver, 1988, p. 1053). Because of these weaknesses noted, and others, we will show later in this chapter that the ADA provides little barrier to the present approach to the rationing of heart transplants under Medicare.

The Age Discrimination in Employment Act. One final insight into the present Supreme Court's reasoning on issues of age discrimination and statutory interpretation was a case decided in 1989, *Public Employees Retirement System of Ohio v. Betts* (hereafter *Betts*, 1989). This case is the Court's most recent interpretation of the meaning of the Age Discrimination in Employment Act of 1967.

The Court considered whether the Public Employees Retirement System of Ohio (PERS) was in conflict with the ADEA. PERS was challenged because it provided that persons under 60 could retire and, if disabled, choose disability benefits rather than retirement benefits. Disability benefits were higher than retirement benefits and provided a minimum payment of at least 30 percent of the retiree's final average salary. Retirement benefits had no corresponding financial floor in Ohio's pension system. Those over 60 who retired because of disability were restricted to the more meager general retirement benefits. The pension plan provided that "once an individual retires on either age-and-service or disability retirement benefits, he or she continues to receive that type of benefit throughout retirement, regardless of age" (*Betts*, 1989, p. 2858).

The plaintiff asserted that this provision denied benefits to her and to other employees on account of age. The court disagreed and held that the plan was constitutional under section 4 (f) (2) of the ADEA, which exempts any "bona fide employees benefit plan such as a retirement, pension, or insurance plan, which is not a subterfuge to evade the purposes of [the act]" (*Betts*, 1989, p. 2860). A bona fide benefit plan is exempt from the purview of the ADEA so long as the plan is not a method of discriminating in other non-fringe-benefit aspects, which would be forbidden by the ADEA's substantive provision. In addition, the *Betts* decision places the burden of the challenge on the employee, who must prove that the challenged benefit plan was intended to serve the purpose of discriminating in a non-fringe-benefit aspect of employment otherwise protected by the ADEA.

On this point, the dissent notes that

> the majority's holding that the employee bears the heavy burden of proving not only that a discriminatory benefit plan implicates non-benefit aspects of employment, but also that it was intended to discriminate, strikes a further blow against the statutory rights of older workers . . . it is one thing for an employee to prove discrimination against older workers. It is considerably more difficult to prove that an employer undertook such discrimination with unlawful motives. (*Betts*, 1989, p. 2871, n. 5)

The court reaffirmed an earlier holding and made clear that "employers may reduce the value of the benefits provided to older workers as necessary to equalize costs for workers of all ages, but they cannot exclude older workers from the coverage of their benefit plans altogether" (*Betts*, 1989, p. 2862). Moreover, the Court said that employers need not show a cost-based justification for age-related differences in benefits, as the ADEA nowhere requires this. The Court stated that under its "construction of the statute, Congress left the employee benefit battle for another day, and legislated only as to hiring and firing, wages and salaries, and other nonfringe-benefit terms and conditions of employment" (p. 2866).

The Court later added that this result permits employers wide latitude in structuring employee benefit plans. Needless to say, pension-related health plans for retirees are one of the major channels through which health care for elderly Americans is financed. The sort of health care that elderly persons receive depends upon the combination of private insurance, pension payments, retiree health benefits, personal resources, and government benefits. For many older persons, retirement health benefits have a tremendous impact on the extent of access to medical care. If employers are permitted to scale those benefits down for older workers, they can effectively reduce the private sector's support for the health care of aged workers who are disabled and/or retired. If the government does not act to counterbalance such a reduction it cannot be charged with rationing, but rather with approving a plan whose end result would be to effectively limit care. If the government allows the private sector to reduce its support for health care plans and does not act to provide added benefits to counteract those reductions, it has effectively permitted rationing for that population.

The Impact of Case Contexts: The Groups Affected, the Interest Affected, and the Medicare Program

If neither the Constitution nor federal statutes provide a fail-safe bulwark against age-based rationing, must we conclude that the road to such rationing is unobstructed? Such a conclusion would be premature. Case law, especially in the constitutional arena, is founded on and intimately shaped by the particular facts and circumstances and the social as well as the legal implications of the case before the Supreme Court. The prospect of age-based rationing of health care thrusts before us variables that have not been considered by the Court in previous cases.

Any official scheme for age-based rationing would likely possess three unique characteristics that could fundamentally alter its constitutional implications. The first characteristic is the nature of the *group affected* under such a scheme. Unlike the statute contested in *Murgia*, which affected healthy state troopers aged 50 and older, a rationing scheme would affect *sick* old people. The second characteristic is that the *interest affected* would be access to health care, not access to employment. Although health care has not been considered a fundamental right for constitutional purposes, it nevertheless carries weightier social implications than any right to employment, especially when, as we have already discussed, that care may be life-sustaining in nature. And the third characteristic is that a rationing scheme would necessarily take place within the *specific context of the Medicare program*, a program in which virtually all elderly Americans participate.

The group affected and the interest affected. The first two characteristics would strike most directly at the "suspect class" analysis under an equal protection claim. The narrow holding in *Murgia* was only that "the class of uniformed state police officers over 50" does not constitute a suspect class (1976, p. 2567). Had older persons in need of medical care and over some age limit—say 75 years of age—imposed by rationing stood before the Court, the Court's equal protection analysis might have tilted toward greater scrutiny.

An instructive case here is the 1985 decision *Cleburne v. Cleburne Living Center* (1985), which struck down a city zoning ordinance requiring a special use permit for group homes for the mentally retarded but not for any other type of residential care facility or multiple dwelling. It demonstrated the Court's willingness to shift its analysis toward strict scrutiny under certain circumstances, while disavowing the existence of a suspect class. The majority of the Court declined to characterize the mentally retarded as a suspect class, or even a "quasi-suspect" class, for purposes of traditional equal protection analysis; nor did the court find a fundamental right to housing or an ability to live in a particular neighborhood at stake. Therefore, the Court purported to apply the highly deferential rational basis test in this instance. Surprisingly, however, the Court went on to scrutinize the rationale and the reasonableness of the ordinance with remarkable thoroughness and intensity, ultimately invalidating it for its constitutional flaws.

The analysis was quite uncharacteristic of the usual hands-off rational basis test, so much so that five members of the Court, concurring in the result, criticized the Court for maintaining a facade of two-tiered analysis of equal protection claims. Two justices, speaking through Justice Stevens, articulated a single rational basis test, which examines in all cases whether "an impartial lawmaker cold logically believe that the classification would serve a legitimate public purpose that transcends the harm to the members of the disadvantaged class" (*Cleburne*, 1985, p. 3261). Justice Marshall, speaking for three of the justices, advocated the sliding-scale type of analysis, described as follows:

> The level of scrutiny employed in an equal protection case should vary with "the constitutional and societal importance of the interest adversely affected and the recognized invidiousness of the basis upon which the particular classification is drawn." (*Cleburne*, 1985, p. 3265)

Clearly, despite the labels applied, equal protection analysis is not a cut-and-dried exercise in which plaintiff groups and plaintiffs' interest at stake are simply sorted into one box or another. In the words of Justice Marshall;

> Permissible distinctions between persons must bear a reasonable relationship to their *relevant* characteristics ... that some retarded people have reduced capacities in some areas does not justify using retardation as a proxy for reduced capacity in areas where relevant individual variations in capacity do exist." (*Cleburne*, 1985, p. 3269)

The same considerations would apply if an age-based rationing scheme were evaluated under equal protection criteria. The question would have to be answered whether age in itself can reasonably be used as a proxy for allocating certain medical resources. *Cleburne* at least makes clear that the Court has been willing to probe such questions, even though the extent to which it would do so remains unclear (Destro, 1986).

The context of the Medicare program. The third characteristic—that a rationing scheme would operate under Medicare—adds an increasingly important new dimension to any equal protection analysis. More and more, the federal government, by means of Medicare, monopolizes and controls health care delivery to the elderly, and its financing. The impact of the Medicare program extends well beyond the program's boundaries, also influencing the nature, the availability, and the cost of private insurance for elderly persons. The predominant form of private health insurance for the elderly—"medigap insurance"—is directly keyed to services not reimbursed by Medicare. This private insurance may cover some of the expenses that Medicare does not, but it remains constrained by the underlying Medicare structure, which limits coverage to only those services deemed "medically necessary" by the Medicare program.

In recent years, Medicare has also exercised an increasing amount of direct control over the private health care sector. For example, Medicare amendments since 1982 have required employers to offer their employees (and employees' spouses) who are 65 and older the same group health plans that are offered to younger workers; imposed limits on the maximum allowable charges for services rendered to Medicare patients by physicians who do *not* participate in Medicare; and required that nonparticipating physicians refund to Medicare beneficiaries any payments collected for services not considered reasonable or necessary under Medicare criteria (Deficit Reduction Act, 1984; Omnibus Reconciliation Act, 1986; Tax Equity and Fiscal Responsibility Act, 1982). Federal control over the full spectrum of health care available to elderly persons is likely to expand if fiscal pressures and demands for long-term care and universal health care coverage continue to grow.

The significance of these changes in health care entitlements for the elderly is that they may affect the "fundamental interest" query required under the equal protection clause and under a related constitutional provision, the due process clauses of the Fifth and Fourteenth Amendments. Applying to the federal and state governments, respectively, these amendments mandate that no person shall be deprived "of life, liberty, or property, without due process of law." Generally, equal protection analysis is used to determine the constitutional validity of the initial classifications used in legislation. Due process analysis is most relevant in adjudicating deprivations of existing rights, whether constitutionally created rights or statutorily created rights.

For example, there is no statutorily recognized right to welfare benefits (*Dandridge v. Williams*, 1970), but if a statutory entitlement is created, certain procedural due process obligations arise to protect beneficiaries who may be deprived of that entitlement (*Goldberg v. Kelly*, 1970).

The Supreme Court recently reaffirmed its view that

the Due Processes Clauses generally confer no affirmative right to governmental aid, even where such aid may be necessary to secure life, liberty, or property interest of which the government itself may not deprive the individual." (*Webster*, 1989, p. 3051)

The Supreme Court has followed this view in holding that the due process clause imposes no duty on a state to provide adequate child protective services (*DeShaney v. Winnebago County*, 1989), in upholding a state welfare regulation that withholds payments for nontherapeutic abortions (*Maher v. Roe*, 1977), and in upholding a congressional amendment to the Medicaid program withholding federal funds for abortions except where the mother's life is endangered (*Harris v. McRae*, 1980).

In each of these cases, the Court characterized the protection of the due process clause as "protection against unwarranted government interference," and not as mandating specific governmental aid (*DeShaney*, 1989, p. 1004). In the abortion cases, the Court relied heavily on the fact that Medicaid was not the only option for securing the health services sought by plaintiffs. The plaintiffs, all poor pregnant women, were not precluded by government action from going out and paying privately for their abortion.

The question of elderly persons' access to health care under Medicare, however, is unique because of the universal nature of the program and its growing control over virtually all health care options for elderly Americans. Since the federal government has so thoroughly undertaken to control the field of health care for the elderly, it has created for beneficiaries an emergent liberty and property interest in the program. Denials of access to care are likely to be held to greater procedural due process protections. The end result of imposing greater due process protection would be similar to that of applying a stricter level of scrutiny under equal protection analysis. Under stricter scrutiny, age as a criterion for rationing could very well be struck down because of its own imprecision, for it excludes from essential benefits those who, while chronologically old, may benefit medically to the same extent as younger persons.

The heterogeneity of the older population is recognized more widely today than ever before. For example, in its report *Life Sustaining Technologies and the Elderly*, the U.S. Congress, Office of Technology Assessment stated clearly that

OTA recognizes and emphasizes, however, that defining the elderly population on the basis of any chronological age criterion tends to mask the heterogeneity of that population. It is inappropriate for clinical decisionmakers or public policymakers to lump together all elderly persons who become candidates for life-sustaining technologies. Rather, the life-threatened elderly should be seen as individuals with widely varying physical and mental status. (1987, pp. 5–6)

Given these acknowledgments, and similar ones that have appeared in medical literature, it becomes increasingly doubtful that rationing on the basis of age could meet either procedural due process requisites or equal protection scrutiny.

Rationing: Does It and Can It Legally Exist at Present?

In 1986 the Supreme Court decided a case involving the care of an imperiled newborn and held that "handicapped infants are entitled to 'meaningful access' to medical services provided by hospitals, and . . . a hospital rule or state policy denying or limiting such access [is] subject to challenge under 504 [of the federal Rehabilitation Act]" (*Bowen v. American Hospital Association*, 1986, p. 2111). This case clearly exposed medical treatment decisions made by health care institutions and their employed or associated providers to scrutiny under section 504 and other protective civil rights statutes (Silver, 1988, p. 994). This case provides an excellent example of the various lenses that can focus on any particular action and the differing legal paths that may subsequently be followed.

In *Bowen*, as might occur in a case involving the nontreatment of an elderly person, the family (in this instance the parents) argued for nontreatment and contended that an acceptance of death was in the "best interest" of the severely handicapped and imperiled newborn. The interveners, beginning with a true stranger who was motivated by a sanctity-of-life philosophy and right-to-life politics, argued that nontreatment was a violation of section 504 of the Rehabilitation Act. The dispute, although couched in statutory language, actually involved a contest between competing world views—and centered on the question of whether any decision to withhold treatment can be a humane and appropriate treatment decision, in the best interests of the patient, or whether it is necessarily a discriminatory action and a form of denying access to care. This case reflects the continuing clash between the proponents of the sanctity-of-life philosophy and the advocates of a quality-of-life analysis.

In this country, there is some historical experience and there are some new ventures involving the rationing of "scarce" and "expensive" care. The distinction between the two is critical. Care is scarce when there are insufficient numbers of machines, transplant organs, or trained staff to meet the demands. Care is expensive when its cost is great.

When dialysis was in its infancy, the intervention was scarce: only a few machines existed, and these were not sufficient to service the mass of patients with renal failure. By its very nature, a scarce resource demands a rationing scheme, that is, an allocation plan. Such rationing is different from the kind considered here, which is the deliberate denial of otherwise available treatment to some individuals who might benefit from it, not because of scarcity but because of expense (Besharov and Silver, 1987). This latter sort of rationing is actually the decision to deny a certain category of people access to care.

As noted, the early history of dialysis involved rationing this new, scarce, life-saving technology. Different localities adopted different means of deciding who should receive the care and who should not. Seattle created a "God squad"—an anonymous committee to weigh the social worth criteria and decide on the relative value of lives. In contrast, Los Angeles County–University of Southern California Medical Center used a lottery (Silver, 1988, p. 999).

When Congress confronted the problem, and a dialysis patient was wheeled onto the floor of the legislature, it rejected any form of rationing and expanded Medicare coverage to provide payment for kidney dialysis for all patients in need. The cost estimates for the program were in the millions; it now costs over $1.5 billion per year (Silver, 1988, p. 1000). This is an example of explicit nonrationing, which, scholars predict, Congress will never again permit.

The most relevant recent example of rationing is the decision as to whether the Medicare program would cover heart transplantation. This was not a congressional decision; rather, it was one arrived at by complex regulations. The program was initially reluctant to extend coverage, perhaps because of its recent sobering experience with the costs of the dialysis program. After a national study that determined that heart transplant programs were no longer experimental and were achieving a high rate of success, and after positive recommendations by special advisory committees, Medicare finally decided in 1987 to extend reimbursement for heart transplantation to Medicare patients (Silver, 1988, pp. 1002–1003).

This Medicare ruling, however, masked a clear policy of denying or discouraging access to this care. The agency placed limits on the eligibility of patients. To qualify for Medicare coverage for a heart transplant, a patient must have been receiving disability benefits under Social Security criteria for 24 months (not a requirement for kidney dialysis) and must not be otherwise disqualified because of "seriously adverse factors," such as older age. A patient over 50 must have an "adequately young physiologic age," no coexisting disease, and no history of behavior or psychiatric illness that might interfere with the rigorous postsurgical medical regimen (Besharov and Silver, 1987, p. 316).

In addition, Medicare restricted the reimbursement of heart transplantation to hospitals with programs which had been in existence since 1985 and had performed a specific number of prior transplants with high survival rates, and which had substantial economic backup for their program and adequate patient selection criteria. In effect, most people over 50 will be excluded; others will be screened out by the medical criteria or will die within the 24 months. Moreover, only approximately 10 hospitals in the nation even qualify for Medicare funding under these regulations (Besharov and Silver, 1987, p. 517). Medicare officials have thus constructed an easily enforceable limit on the possible number of heart transplants. They have effectively rationed this expensive and scarce health care intervention, although it is used beneficially for some older patients (see chapter 3, above).

Perspectives on the Future

Health care for elderly persons could be rationed in any number of ways: officially and directly by congressional or by state legislative action; indirectly by federal or state regulation; or haphazardly by institutional policies and/or by individual physicians' decisions designed to maximize income, minimize loss, and avoid legal issues. This list progresses from the most visible and clearly evident mechanism to those forms of rationing least accessible to public scrutiny and review. The nature of a legal challenge and its prospects for success would depend, in the first instance, on the rationing method chosen.

It is simply not certain whether an explicit rationing scheme using old age as a criterion and adopted either by Congress or by a state legislature could survive a challenge based on equal protection arguments, especially if the Supreme Court were to expand its suspect class analysis or otherwise be moved to impose a higher level of scrutiny. An ADA challenge to congressional action would be ineffective, as specific legislative formulations are exempt from scrutiny under the terms of the act.

Perhaps the best protection from the denial of life-sustaining care may lie in assertions by elderly persons of a "fundamental interest" in such care, due to the growing universality of the Medicare program and their reliance on it. This possible protection, however, is politically fragile. Congress could amend or even repeal Medicare if it so chose. The repeal of the major provisions of the Medicare Catastrophic Coverage Act is but the most recent evidence of this ability. However, this same example also illustrates the impact some older constituents can have in determining the future of Medicare.

The state of Oregon and Alameda County, California, have recently enacted regulations limiting the access of Medicaid beneficiaries to organ transplants (*Health Advocate*, 1989). In some well-publicized cases individuals have died, yet the policies remain in effect. The survival of these policies under the scrutiny of the public and the press gives some notion of their political strength. It also contradicts the statement of conventional wisdom, often offered, that politicians will pass legislation compromising "statistical lives" but not "individuals' lives" (Mehlman, 1985, p. 254). The rationing of specific advanced technological interventions places dying poor people in the spotlight. However, the legislation has survived and the people have not.

The most likely and the most troubling scenario projects that rationing will be carried out by an allocation process concealed from public view, a so-called responsible system of allocation implemented inconspicuously by private institutions and practitioners. This sort of rationing will be difficult to uncover and even more difficult to prove and prevent. It will respond to implied regulatory messages from Medicare and Medicaid; it will react to reimbursement formulas and market reward. Most worrisome, it will couch personal and institutional prejudice in the language of medical and quasiscientific criteria.

In our multitiered system of health care, the individuals most likely to be affected by such informal rationing and allocation patterns will be poor people and members of minority groups. Individual tort suits to contest these decisions will be difficult to mount, as tort lawyers generally work on a contingent fee basis and the recovery—a measure of lost earnings—will likely be low in such cases.

The lack of accountability, the random nature of decisions, and the lack of any check upon the personal preferences and prejudices of the health care providers all argue against encouraging these hidden mechanisms. The principles of equity and justice in a free society demand that we arrive at these difficult decisions openly and, by so doing, confront ourselves and our political representatives with our assumptions about aging and about the value of aged persons' lives.

References

Age Discrimination Act (1975). Public Law 94-135, as amended, codified at 42 U.S.C., 6101 et seq.

Age Discrimination in Employment Act (1967). Public Law 90-202, as amended, codified at 29 U.S.C., sec. 621 et seq.

American Bar Assocation (1987). Legal problems of the elderly, report no. 106B. In *Summary of the House of Delegates: 1987 annual meeting, San Francisco, California, August 11–12, 1987*, pp. 14–18. Chicago: American Bar Association.

American Bar Association (1989a). *Guardianship: an agenda for reform.* Washington, D.C.: American Bar Association, Commission on the Mentally Disabled, and Commission on Legal Problems of the Elderly.

American Bar Association (1989b). Mentally disabled, report no. 104. In *Summary of action of the House of Delegates: 1989 midyear meeting, Denver, Colorado, February 6–7, 1989*, pp. 22–32.

American Bar Association, Commission on Legal Problems of the Elderly, and National Judicial College (1986). *Statement of recommended judicial practices.* Washington, D.C.: American Bar Association, Commission on Legal Problems of the Elderly.

Associated Press (1987). *Guardians of the elderly: an ailing system.* Special report. New York: Associated Press.

Besharov, D.J., and Silver, J.D. (1987). Rationing access to advanced medical techniques. *Journal of Legal Medicine,* 8(4), 507–532.

Bolling v. Sharpe (1954). 74 S.Ct. 693.

Bowen v. American Hospital Association (1986). 106 S.Ct. 2101.

Brakel, S.J. (1985). Historical trends. In S.J. Brakel, J. Parry, and B.A. Weiner, *The mentally disabled and the law* (3rd ed.). Chicago: American Bar Foundation.

Cleburne v. Cleburne Living Center (1985). 105 S.Ct. 3249.

Cruzan v. Director, Missouri Department of Health (1990). 110 S.Ct. 2841.

Dandridge v. Williams (1970). 90 S.Ct. 1153.

Deficit Reduction Act (1984). Public Law 98-369.

DeShaney v. Winnebago County Department of Social Services (1989). 109 S.Ct. 998.

Destro, R.A. (1986). Quality-of-life ethics and constitutional jurisprudence: the demise of national rights and equal protection for the disabled and incompetent. *Journal of Contemporary Health Law and Policy,* 2, 71–130.

Deutsch, A. (1949). *The mentally ill in America: a history of their case and treatment from colonial times* (2nd ed.). New York: Columbia University Press.

Estelle v. Gamble (1976). 97 S.Ct. 285.

Evans, W.D. (1977). Massachusetts v. Murgia: a fifty-year-old policeman and traditional equal protection analysis—are they both past their prime? *Pepperdine Law Review,* 4, 369–387.

Frontiero v. Richardson (1973). 93 S.Ct. 1764.

Frosberg, B.B. (1986). Advanced age as a measure of capacity and competency. *BIFOCAL,* 7(2), 4–6. Washington, D.C.: American Bar Association, Commission on Legal Problems of the Elderly.

Goldberg v. Kelly (1970). 90 S.Ct. 1011.

Harris v. McRae (1980). 100 S.Ct. 2671.

Health Advocate (1989). Rationing medical services begins in Oregon and California. No. 160, Spring, p. 3.

In re Eichner (1981). 52 N.Y.2d 363; also 420 N.E.2d 64, *cert. denied*, 454 U.S. 858.

In re Fisher (1989). *New York Law Journal*, September 8, p. 2.

In re Quinlan (1976). 70 N.J. 10; also 355 A.2d 647.

In re Storer (1981). 52 N.Y.2d 363; also 420 N.E.2d 64, *cert. denied*, 454 U.S. 858.

In re Westchester County Medical Center ex rel O'Connor (1988). 534 N.Y.S.2d 886; also 72 N.Y.2d 517, 531 N.E.2d 607.

Kirshenbaum, S.M. (1977). Law note: defeat of the constitutional challenge to mandatory retirement, Massachusetts Board of Retirement v. Murgia. *Toledo Law Review, 8,* 764–783.

Maher V. Roe (1977). 97 S.Ct. 2376.

Massachusetts Board of Retirement v. Murgia (1976). 96 S.Ct. 2562.

Mehlman, M.J. (1985). Rationing expensive lifesaving medical treatments. *Wisconsin Law Review, 2,* 239–278.

Omnibus Reconciliation ACt (1986). Public Law 96-735, enacted August 13, 1981, as amended.

Parry, J. (1985). Incompetency, guardianship, and restoration. In S.J. Brakel, J. Parry, and B.A. Weiner, eds., *The mentally disabled and the law* (3rd ed.). Chicago: American Bar Foundation.

Public Employees Retirement System of Ohio v. Betts (1989). 109 S.Ct. 2854.

Rehabilitation Act (1973). Public Law 93-122, as amended, 1982, codified at 29 U.S.C. 794.

Rotunda, R.D., Nowak, J.E., and Young, J.N. (1986). *Treatise on constitutional law: substantive and procedure,* vol. 2. Saint Paul, Minn.: West Publishing Co.

San Antonio School District v. Rodriguez (1973). 93 S.Ct. 2266.

Schmidt, W., Miller, K., Bell, W., and New, B. (1981). *Public guardianship and the elderly.* Cambridge, Mass.: Ballinger Publishing Co.

Silver, J.D. (1988). From Baby Doe to Grandpa Doe: the impact of the federal Age Discrimination Act on the "hidden rationing of medical care." *Catholic University Law Review, 37,* 993–1072.

Society for the Right to Die (1988). *The physician and the hopelessly ill patient; legal, medical and ethical guidelines,* 1988 suppl. New York: Society for the Right to Die.

Spring, J.C., and Dubler, N.N. (1990). *Conservatorship in New York State: does it serve the needs of the elderly?* A report of the Committee on Legal Problems of the Aging. *The Record,* Association of the Bar of the City of New York, vol. 45, no. 3.

Superintendent of Belchertown State School v. Saikewicz (1978). 373 Mass. 728; also 370 N.E.2d 417.

Tax Equity and Fiscal Responsibility Act (1982). Public Law 97-248.

U.S. Congress, Office of Technology Assessment (1987). *Life-sustaining technologies and the elderly.* Washington, D.C.: U.S. Government Printing Office.

Webster v. Missouri (1989). 109 S.Ct. 3040.

Weiner, B.A. (1985). Treatment rights. In S.J. Brakel, J. Parry, and B.A. Weiner, eds., *The mentally disabled and the law* (3rd ed.). Chicago: American Bar Foundation.

Youngberg v. Romero (1982). 102 S.Ct. 2452.

6

Justice for Elderly People in Jewish and Christian Thought

STEPHEN G. POST, Ph.D.

Proposals to deny life-saving treatment on the basis of age violate the moral thrust of both Judaism and Christianity. Ordinarily, the term *Judeo-Christian* is to be avoided because it assumes broad continuities between Judaism and Christianity when in fact major disparities exist, but when discussing their common ground, age-neutral theories of justice, the term *Judeo-Christian* is entirely appropriate. Both traditions protest against all theories of justice that would discriminate against individuals on the basis of age.

In the Judeo-Christian tradition, justice is held to apply equally to all, regardless of age. Because young persons and old persons are often vulnerable due to their dependence on others, this tradition places particular emphasis on their needs. Both the old widow and the young orphan have their just claims, preached the Hebrew prophets, and the one is not to be pitted against the other. The Holiness Code (Lev. 19), a cornerstone of Jewish ethics, requires that orphans, blind people, deaf people, and elderly people be given special care. Christian social thought deviated not one iota from Jewish thought in this regard. With particular firmness, Jewish and Christian ethics oppose injustice toward human beings who are at the beginning of life's journey or in the fullness of years, for at these edges of life human vulnerability is greatest, and inhumanity is most likely to surface.

The Function of Religious Ethics

Before explicating how the Judeo-Christian vision of justice acts as a stalwart alternative to recent proposals for the age-based rationing of

120

health care, it is important to stress briefly that this ethical vision has major social significance.

Religious ethics can be appreciated as a set of reasonable moral restraints without which social harmonies would be destroyed. Such harmonies are made more firm for society through their expression in religious narratives and symbols. As the nineteenth-century French sociologist Emil Durkheim (1965) maintained, religion and religious ethics are in large part projections of the values required for social prosperity.

Accordingly, throughout this chapter, religious ethics are interpreted not as arbitrary divine commands but as rational norms established over time by communities and expressed in symbolic forms. Indeed, the assumption that religious ethics are "irrational" or "antirational" has largely given way to the framework suggested by philosopher Ernst Cassirer (1944), who viewed the creation of symbols in myth, art, and religion as creative human attempts to deal with problems of meaning and value.

Underlying religious expressions of ethics, one often discovers the dictates of practical moral reasoning. Thus, Jewish ethicist Ronald M. Green writes:

> Whatever their specific teachings, religions agree on the basic rules of morality. All prohibit wanton killing or injury of other persons (although many permit legitimate self-defense); all condemn deception and the breaking of solemn promises. On the positive side, all require giving some minimum of aid to those in need; all require reparation for wrongs committed; and all ask some expression of gratitude for assistance received. (1988, p. 11)

If religious ethics are associated with "basic rules of morality," as Green suggests, then even the secular ethicist can discern something of rational value in the age-neutrality of Judeo-Christian justice. Those who adhere to Judaism or Christianity will not require the above rationalist interpretation of the precepts of their religion. Indeed, approximately 90 percent of Americans are religious, and a significant fraction are Jewish, while the vast majority are Christian (Gallop, 1981).

The Jewish Tradition

Joseph Cardinal Bernardin articulated the Roman Catholic definition of justice as follows: "We must defend the right to life of the weakest among us; we must also be supportive of the quality of life of the powerless among us: the old and the young, the hungry and the homeless" (1985, p. 38). Bernardin's reference to a grouping of "the old and the young," rather than to separate treatments of the old *or* the young, is fully consistent with the theory of justice characteristic of Jewish thought.

This perspective is evidenced by Hebrew Scripture, in which provision for old people is taken with utmost seriousness. Deuteronomy, for example, brings together widow and orphan in a single passage: "You shall not deprive aliens and orphans of justice nor take a widow's cloak in pledge" (24:17). On the condition of providing for "the alien, the orphan, and the widow," the Israelites will be blessed by their God in all that they undertake (Deut. 24:19). Not all widows are old, but Jewish tradition has taken these passages to have special significance for the way elderly persons are treated. To encourage the fulfillment of these moral duties, God reminds the Israelites of their suffering in Egypt as slaves before the Exodus (Deut. 24:22).

Application of the Exodus metaphor to the plight of elderly persons has a perennial significance. Michael Walzer highlights "the great presence and power in Western political thought" of "the idea of a deliverance from suffering and oppression" as it is articulated in the Exodus account (1985, p. ix). It would be difficult to find a set of passages more influential for Western morals than those pertaining to the Exodus from Egypt; and in the context of affirming society's duties toward both the young and the old, the reminder of the Exodus experience is significant for what it says about the importance of these obligations.

In Hebrew Scripture, Exodus 20:12 places the commandment to honor one's father and mother first among those prescriptions dealing with relations among people. Leviticus 19:32 also requires the Israelite to give "honor to the aged." Proverbs 20:29 states, "The glory of young men is their strength, the dignity of old men their gray hairs"; and Proverbs 23:22 requires that the old not be despised. Similar passages abound in the Hebrew Bible, all placed within the context of a larger theological framework of *chesed*, or steadfast covenantal love between a parental deity—presumably a very old one at that—and the "children of Israel."

The Covenant

Indeed, the entire scriptural history of Israel describes the ideal of a restored relationship between Jahweh (God) and the wayward children who reject him. Covenantal mutuality between young and old people is at the very center of Jewish thought, so that any "pragmatic" disregard for aged persons violates a basic norm of reciprocity (see Heschel, 1959).

The duties of reciprocity clearly do not encompass an obligation for older persons to die before life has run its course in order to "benefit" young persons. Some may automatically dismiss the ideal of reciprocity simply because it is ensconced in a theological context. However, even when viewed from the perspective of the cultural anthropologist, this context can be appreciated as the narrative and symbolic setting in which a tribe of people expressed an essential social harmony.

Equality before God

Absolutely central to the Jewish concept of justice is the notion of *imago Dei*, namely, that all persons are made in the image of God. As one interpreter of Judaism writes, "the idea of equality before God and therefore of equality and justice in human relations is found throughout the literature" of Jewish thought (Abernethy, 1959, p. 29).

Because human beings are all equally the creations of Jahweh and all have equal worth based on their relatedness to Jahweh, the value of persons does not ultimately depend on their social usefulness. To be sure, the Hebrews respected elderly persons because those advanced in years can pass wisdom and tradition down to future generations. Even if the capacities of elderly persons should wane so that no social function is possible for them, however, values transcending social function still include the elderly within a circle of moral protection and justice that encompasses all human beings.

A clear moral message of Judaism is that there exists a basic human equality that underlies more superficial inequalities between persons based on qualities such as talent, age, and color. "The Lord is the maker of them all" (Prov. 22:2), and equally the God of all. As the prophet Malachi asked: "Have we not all one father? Did not one God create us? Why do we violate the covenant of our forefathers by being faithless to one another?" (2:10)

The idea of equality, in one form or another, is consistent with all Western political and moral thought. It surely has some of its roots in Greek and Roman thought, particularly that of the Stoics. They identified the human capacity to reason as a link with God, and thereby attributed to each human being a spark of divinity. However, Judaism goes further than Stoicism and other ancient philosophies by developing a theory of equality independent of any innate human capacity. Differences in capacities, age, and the like have no relevance to Jahweh's concern with his creatures. Thus, the Hebrew prophets taught the ideal of a reign of equality under divine justice and righteousness. The influence of these religious origins, transmitted largely through Christianity, is preserved in Western law and in American political institutions.

Theological context or no, this basic human equality remains a worthy moral aspiration. It was translated by the Enlightenment philosopher Kant (1964) into the strictly rationalist doctrine of "respect for persons," and holds a major place in modern ethical thought. Whether this ideal of equality can be sustained in the absence of a theological center of gravity is one of the challenges confronting our aging society.

Justice for Widows

Before turning to Christian thought on justice, some attention is due the Jewish emphasis on meeting the needs of the vulnerable old widow. Among the very old in contemporary American society, women far outnumber men. It has been estimated that in the United States, by the year 2000, there will be 37.2 men for every 100 women aged 85 and older (Riley and Riley, 1986, p. 66). If women continue to outlive men, even higher percentages of the very old will be women. Hence, to a significant degree, the discussions about age-based rationing of health care concern the fate of old women.

Without overemphasizing the gender dimension of the question of justice for elderly persons, it can be said that the issue is not entirely gender-neutral. Already, researchers have begun to address the health and economic status of older women. The themes taken up range from feminism and anti-ageism to elderly women and poverty (Herzog et al., 1989). A cross-cultural treatment of the experiences of widows has recently been the subject of a two-volume study (Lopata, 1987).

However much Judaism can be chastised for its patriarchal elements, the tradition must be credited for its concern for the care of the elderly widow. The vulnerable widow is firmly encompassed within the sphere of justice. Should harm befall her, the covenant with Jahweh has been broken and his blessing is thereby revoked.

The "Length of Days"

It is fitting to close this discussion of the Jewish prophetic tradition with David M. Feldman's affirmation of "length of days" as a blessing for observing the laws of the Torah (1986, p. 97). In summarizing the Jewish respect for age and the wisdom associated with it, Feldman asserts that Judaism categorically rejects materialistic and utilitarian evaluations of elderly persons. As he writes;

> If, among other things, the human soul is the repository of one's feelings, experiences, memories and the like, then the older the person the greater the capacity of the soul. The opposite point of view judges a person by his productivity, by what or how much he or she can produce and contribute to economic or social life. But this materialistic valuation, we are taught, must be avoided in favor of a spiritual yardstick that judges one for what he is rather than for what he does. (p. 98)

Thus does Judaism reject the negative images of the elderly that arise from cultural overemphasis on the virtues of being young, productive in the workplace, and independent. Growing old in contemporary America, as Robert N. Butler suggests, "is an affront to a culture with a passion for youth and productive capacity" (1975, p. xi). Judaism offers an alternative view of the elderly person, one subject neither to the vicissitudes of shifting social circumstances nor to the tyranny of the "normal" as contemporary American culture defines it.

Christian Thought

Christian social thought is, from its earliest beginnings, continuous with Jewish philosophy on issues concerned with aging. The earliest and most valuable surviving piece of Christian literature other than the New Testament is a letter written circa A.D. 96 by Clement of Rome to the sister church at Corinth (see Staniforth, 1968, p. 17). As a moral counsel, the Epistle of Clement reads thus: "Leave off wickedness, and learn to do right. Seek justice, relieve the oppressed, do right by the fatherless, act fairly to the widow" (p. 27). In a similar but slightly later document, the Epistle of Barnabas, written before A.D. 132, the "way of the darkness" includes arrogance, duplicity, manslaughter, greed, and a host of other vices. Of those who follow this way, it is said that "the widow and the orphan are nothing to them" (p. 219).

Protecting Vulnerable Persons: Young and Old

In these and other early Christian epistles, the concern is more with practice than with dogma; and abandoning the vulnerable, whether very young or very old, is anathema. This crucial theme in the tradition of prophetic justice was taken by Christianity from Judaism, and was continued through centuries of Western culture. Thus did the medieval Church take upon itself the special mission of protecting those persons who are at the beginning and the end of life (Cadoux, 1925, pp. 596–610). Regarding the elderly, 1 Timothy, a letter included in the New Testament canon, sums up the ideal of harmony between young and old aptly: "Never be harsh with an elder; appeal to him as if he were your father. Treat the younger men as brothers, the older women as mothers, and the younger as your sisters, in all purity" (5:1–2).

Saint Augustine, writing in the early fifth century A.D. about the tranquility in the peaceful City of God, stressed the importance of beneficence toward aged persons (Augustine, 1950). Thomas Aquinas echoed this theme, as did the theologians of the Protestant Reformation. The first duties of charity are toward those in society who are most likely to be treated unjustly.

The Primacy of Need

Christian social thought is, like Jewish social thought, remarkable for its unwillingness to place needy persons in competition with one another for the essential goods and services without which human beings cannot prosper. The moral logic behind this unwillingness is related to the prophetic suspicion that human greed and avarice inevitably underlie any assertion that some truly needy persons must regrettably be subjected to destruction inflicted by distributive injustice. Justice addresses the disparity between rich and poor, and refuses to pit poor against poor. It is the will to power and the human propensity for exploitation that undergird the convenient device of placing persons with genuine needs in opposing corners, for example, "young *versus* old."

David P. Barash argues that the contemporary Western mind is "caught in a conflicting cross fire of intellectual traditions" (1983, p. 6). The Greco-Roman view of aging as a great misfortune is in tension with the Jewish and Christian tendency to emphasize the positive aspects of growing old. Consistent with the Greco-Roman view, cultural anthropologists can cite evidence of tribes in which elder persons, as they became unable to pull their weight, were "likely to be neglected, abandoned, or even killed outright" (Barash, 1983, p. 178), due in part to the difficulty of primitive life. However, as anthropologist Leo W. Simmons pointed out, the more likely scenario in early civilizations was one in which "the aged, along with other dependents, have found some reliable assurance of support . . . in the most advanced societies—such as the Inca or Aztec—[this is provided] through organized systems of old-age assistance" (1945, p. 26).

Nevertheless, it remains true that some societies had and do have moral blind spots with regard to the respect due all persons regardless of age. Societies influenced by Judeo-Christian thought at least possess an ability to see dignity regardless of age, and therefore represent moral progress in an often morally ambiguous world. Such progress, though, is fragile; it is a thin veneer over the potential chaos of exploitation and destruction. The reported killing by four Austrian nurse's aides of a possible 49 elderly persons in a long-term care setting in 1989 highlights this fragility (Protzman, 1989, p. 1).

Rationing and Equality

Proposals that health care be rationed on the basis of age weaken the thin veneer of equality. They segregate elderly persons into a separate category: the category of those who, because they have lived out most of their productive years, are no longer encompassed by justice in quite the same way that others are. The basic equality found in Judeo-Christian thought is thus weakened by theories of justice that, even if not meant to do so, contribute to the isolation and the vulnerability of a particular age group.

Those who advocate the categorical denial of life-saving care to older persons as a matter of public policy contend that such a policy will not erode time-honored standards of equality. Bioethicist Daniel Callahan argues that by providing elderly persons with basic long-term care rather than life-sustaining cures, society fulfills its obligations in a manner consistent with respect for persons (1987, p. 151; 1990, pp. 151–154). If hospicelike care alone were provided, contends Callahan, the elderly would still be treated with full equality and dignity.

However, the separation of elderly persons into a category of those eligible only for hospicelike care would likely contribute to a spirit of inequality rather than one of equality. Such categorization would send a message: elderly persons do not have the same rights as others, and are unworthy of those forms of care generally used to save lives. Categorically denying elderly persons access to life-saving treatments from which they would benefit (e.g., survive for a significant period of time with an acceptable quality of life) would initiate a dangerous process of ghettoization.

Once this process begins, where will it end? The theories upholding age-based rationing systematically omit reference to the human propensity for gross inhumanity. The abyss of discrimination is too easily justified by reference to the expedient. If the twentieth century has taught us anything, it is that all such forms of categorization must be nipped in the bud. Ethics is less about achieving the *summum bonum* than about avoiding the *summum malum*. As the political realists know well, its major concern is with placing fences around the abyss. Proposals for age-based rationing may have a certain abstract appeal; but within the realistic context of human callousness and injustice, such proposals could usher in demographic holocaust. Those who formulate and promulgate such proposals surely mean well; their intentions are probably beyond reproach. But the road to moral catastrophe is paved with good intentions.

Rationing and Freedom

Like equality, human freedom is an ideal that has deep roots in Judeo-Christian thought, although in practice, society may frequently have fallen short of the ideal. According to Jewish thought, nothing is more sinful than the idolatrous worship of political rulers; monotheism deprived rulers of their former claims to divinity, so that the authority of rulers could henceforth never be more than penultimate. Regarding Christianity, it can be said that Jesus refused all power but the power of love. As theologian Nicholas Berdyaev wrote, "Truth nailed upon the cross compels nobody, oppresses no one; it must be accepted and confessed freely" (1957, p. 197).

No matter at what age the cutoff point were to be set, should elderly persons be denied various treatments simply because they are old? Not only would such a practice violate the fragile moral ideal of human equality, it would violate the equally fragile ideal of human freedom.

On behalf of freedom, it must be affirmed that no individual should have to die knowing that his or her life was needlessly stripped of years of good-quality existence. Although the moral balance between individual and society sometimes requires that the latter hold sway, any societal imposition on a matter so private and subjectively monumental as an individual's sense that it is not yet time to die is surely unacceptable. While society has no obligation to prolong dying, or to provide interventions that have only a remote possibility of restoring health and longevity, persons who still have good years remaining as a result of intervention have a basic right to treatment, regardless of age.

Demographic data, newly created theories of justice, and suggested "natural life-spans" are intellectually interesting, but they have no clear moral authority over a personal decision to welcome something as ultimate as death. The demands of mutuality between generations do not require of the elderly person a socially coerced downward course through preventable morbidity toward a preventable death. In the final analysis, we must allow the individual conscience its due, and acknowledge the heterogeneity of persons within all age cohorts.

Freedom and "Overtreatment"

To endorse the self-determination of the individual elderly person is not to endorse the overtreatment of those who are dying. The task of medicine does not include extending the life of a patient "well beyond the time at which there is reasonable hope of returning him to a reasonably healthy state" (Kass, 1985, p. 163). However, when the restoration of health is possible, the moral resolve of medicine is to proceed according to the patient's preferences, regardless of his or her age. It is precisely this resolve that ethicists working from within the tradition of clinical healing are reluctant to compromise. As medical ethicist Richard M. Zaner states, "medical practice is guided by the moral resolve of physicians to put their knowledge, experience, time, and talents at the disposal of distressed or damaged persons individually or as groups" (1988, p. 39). It is this resolve to help other people in need, regardless of external social pressures, that is ultimately threatened by the proposals for old-age-based rationing.

Of course, if a treatment is futile, no individual has a claim to it. However, if a treatment offers a reasonable degree of benefit to the patient, then ideally it is he or she who should decide on its use. Perhaps an elderly person will feel that his or her life span is complete, and that any major medical interventions would be wasted. However, respect for persons and for human dignity—notions that transcend age—require that the ground gained for individual conscience not be lost to public policy coercions. A concern for justice in the distribution of health care should inform the conscience of every citizen, including the old, as should awareness of the "right to die."

To live in an open society is to make moral decisions within the context of noncoercive relationships. Freedom respects the individual who refuses restraint because of his or her depth of conscience. Freedom does not allow for herding people together in groups on the basis of their demographic characteristics. In an open society, freedom exerts a moral pressure against authorities who would deter the individual conscience.

Underlying proposals for age-based rationing is a lack of trust in the competence of older persons to make reasonable choices about life and death, futility and benefit. Unfortunately, there is a stereotype that older persons, simply because they are old, do not make sound decisions. They are frequently treated as though they were infantilized, and their rights to autonomy and confidentiality are ignored.

However, older persons, in the absence of serious degrees of incompetence, can make sound decisions; and no decision is more intimate and inaccessible to the outsider than a decision about the use of life-saving treatments. As James F. Childress writes, "It is morally imperative to attend to individual differences, rather than to treat the elderly, even the infirm or sick elderly, as a class" (1984, p. 31).

To propose allocating health care on the basis of age is to forget Aristotle's observation that theories of justice are inexact, and it is to underestimate the creativity of the individual conscience in balancing individual needs with social needs. Finally, it is to presume a level of consensus on this sensitive issue that a pluralistic society cannot approach. There are, after all, subgroups in our society that value elderly individuals even more than young ones because old persons transmit traditional wisdom and are more intertwined in the social experience of a community (Kilner, 1984).

People, especially old people, do need to know that it is all right to die, that there is nothing wrong about deciding to let life run its course. Some might with good reason accept the skeptical attitude toward medical technology and so-called medical progress that informs the rationing proposals. However, these attitudes, if they are to be valid, must be freely accepted rather than imposed. Many people have grown wary of medical heroics at the end of life, and refuse them. Advance directives such as living wills, if widely utilized and properly adhered to by physicians, could in large part solve the problem of overtreatment.

True, it can sometimes be difficult for the individual to overcome the reluctance of contemporary medicine to declare that anyone is, in fact, dying. As pressure for cost containment rises, however, this reluctance of physicians may very well subside. Regardless, although physicians do tend to overtreat dying persons and to make false promises respecting outcomes, these tendencies can be tempered. It is reasonable to expect that medicine can be reformed in these areas, and unreasonable to impose restrictions on treatment for elderly persons as an alternative to such reforms, thereby harming both aged individuals and the practice of medicine.

Self-Determination

The sense that each individual's life-span and biography is mysterious (so to speak), beyond the easy comprehension of outsiders, requires that there be respect for personal choice. It is unfair, then, to assert that there is some age at which "normal" life is biographically complete. Such an assertion may serve the positive purpose of encouraging elderly persons to reflect on mortality and the life cycle. However, this assertion can never be an absolute prescription for the individual, who certainly knows—more reliably than does the best politician or biomedical ethicist—when his or her life is no longer worth saving. The purposes, meanings, and creativities of individuals are too profound, even ineffable, to be treated homogeneously.

On the theme of self-determination, this country's best-known octogenarian ethicist, Joseph Fletcher, provides insight. Long an advocate of the right to die and of mercy killing, Fletcher refuses to embrace the idea of age-based rationing because it implies that the elderly have a "duty to die." Impersonal demographic data are not the criteria upon which Fletcher wants his life ended. Rather, in a properly individualized manner, he intends to decide "when the flame is no longer worth the candle, when it's better to be dead, but not for reasons of social justice" (Fletcher, 1988, p. 3). Death, he contends, should never be imposed on those who are unwilling; better to "take comfort in the knowledge that patients and their families, like people in general, are open more and more to giving death a welcome" (p. 4). This is the optimism that proponents of age-based rationing lack. One might justifiably encourage an elderly person to let go of life "whenever it is in the patient's own best interest," but at no point ought we to allow death to become a matter of socioeconomic policy, contends Fletcher (p. 4).

To fully appreciate the thoughts of those like Fletcher who are themselves old and yet still fell that life is worth living, a brief glimpse of Japanese culture is worthwhile. The fifteenth-century Japanese playwright Zeami Motokiyo wrote a famous *No* drama about an old crone (a withered elderly woman) who was deserted on Mount Obasute in Shinano province. Several travelers encounter the ghost of the old woman, who had been left to die. "How shameful," she cried out, "Long ago I was abandoned here" (Motokiyo, 1977, p. 715). In the same drama, a man named Wada no Hikonaga grows up under the care of this woman, his aunt. From the day of his marriage, his wife hates his aunt and makes accusations against her. Hikonaga does not listen to his wife until, at length, he "[forgets] his aunt's many years of kindness" and bows to his wife's demands. He takes his aunt up to the top of Mount Obasute, "Mountain of the Deserted Old Women." There the aunt dies all alone, still "clinging to the world" and feeling that her life remains unfinished. The drama ends with the ghost lamenting, "Now, alone, deserted, a moss-grown wintry hag" (p. 714). This imagery from fifteenth-century Japan so well captures the way in which the old are morally violated when others determine for them that their life span has ended.

Intergenerational Virtue

Thus far, the focus of this chapter has been on precepts concerning the personal freedom of elderly persons. Such precepts can be complemented by a set of moral dicta that any particular elderly individual might accept or reject.

Ambiguous notions of intergenerational conflict and justice between generations, which have now become common parlance, appear to underlie proposals for age-based rationing (Crystal, 1982; Preston, 1984). This arbitrarily framed conflict between the young and the old may begin to lead American society to forget the moral norm of mutuality and reciprocity between generations that is so deeply embedded in its religious heritages.

Ethicists should discourage the adversarial construct of intergenerational relations by encouraging virtue on the part of both the young and the old. While the importance of filial duties among young people should be addressed, a degree of self-sacrifice and other-regarding love among elderly people—directed both toward the young and toward one another—should also be encouraged.

Many contemporary observers find no fault with narcissistic values among older persons. For instance, Nouwen and Gaffney (1974), in their *Aging: The Fulfillment of Life*, refer repeatedly to old age as "a rainbow of promises." A major exception to this predominant outlook is a recent work by Stephen Sapp, who soundly indicts ethicists for sanctioning self-centeredness in elderly persons:

> How much fuller might old age be if spent in some form of service to others? How much more purpose might be found for the sometimes seemingly endless time if the lost responsibilities of job and children are replaced, not exclusively with *self*-oriented recreational pastimes, but with activities that contribute to the welfare of others? (1987, p. 133)

Ethicists have not seen fit to encourage elderly persons in the direction of beneficence and sacrifice. Sapp counters the mainstream with his claim that older people need to remember that the call to serve others knows no time limit (p. 159). Of course, most elderly persons are other-regarding as much as they are self-regarding, and it is an error to suggest that the old are any less virtuous than other age groups; indeed, the contrary may be the case.

Any reasonable person, and certainly any person steeped in Jewish or Christian thought, will be appalled at the image of conflict between young and old that is now evident. Mutual caring between persons young and old within the community is the valid familial and social ideal, and deviations from it are unfortunate. A pressing question is how to sustain the intergenerational covenant. The meaning of *covenant* has been expressed eloquently by James F. Childress: "'Covenant' suggests a reciprocal relationship in which there is receiving and giving. But it is not reducible to a contract with a specific quid pro quo, for it also contains an element of the gratuitous which cannot be specified" (1982, p. 42). Participants in a covenant must be at least as other-regarding as they are self-regarding, and probably more so.

Elderly persons within the Christian tradition might begin to think about their duties to the young by remembering the high dignity Jesus of Nazareth conferred on children by embracing them and blessing them despite the protests of his disciples, who did not like to see such irritating creatures near their master (Mark 10). Indeed, the Nazarene went so far as to make of the little child a prototype for those who would enter the Kingdom of God. A primary Christian goal of intergenerational relations in an aging society, then, is to encourage the old to nurture the young.

Obligations of Old People to Young People

Somewhat paradoxically, through serving the young, the old help to secure their own well-being. In his classic work of modern anthropology,

Simmons examined the moral status of old people in primitive societies and found that they are highly regarded when they contribute most to the lives of the young: "Perhaps the simplest and most effective way of eliciting the support of others has been to render essential—if possible, indispensable—services to them" (1945, pp. 82–83).

The fact is that the roles assumed by the elderly have in the past "hardly ever been passive." Moreover, their activities have done much to influence their security. Regarding elderly persons among the ancient Hebrews, Simmons writes, "Their security has been more often an achievement than an endowment—an achievement in which favorable opportunities have been matched with active personal accomplishments" (1945, p. 82). These accomplishments were augmented at the onset of old age. Covenantal duties wane only when one can no longer fulfill them, and obligations to one's juniors do not cease when one arrives at some arbitrary age, say 65. When the old break the covenant, they contribute to an unnecessary conflict that can result in their own eventual neglect.

This emphasis on the duties of old persons is intended only as an appeal to personal conscience. There are elderly individuals who will wish to live their lives independent of a covenant with the young. Nevertheless, Jewish and Christian thought recommends that those who are old make a significant effort to nurture those who are young, as well as one another.

Callahan is convinced that elderly persons "cannot claim a right to self-absorption or an exemption from civic duties" (1987, p. 49). He cites a very pointed and morally demanding passage from Cicero:

> Old men . . . as they become less capable of physical exertion, should redouble their intellectual activity, and their principal occupation should be to assist the young, their friends, and above all their country with their wisdom and sagacity. There is nothing they should guard against so much as languor and sloth. Luxury, which is shameful at ever period of life, makes old age hideous. If it is united with sensuality, the evil is twofold. Age thus becomes a disgrace on itself and aggravates the shameless license of the young. (p. 51)

This passage is too stern, and presents a rather narrow image of meaning in old age. However, it provides a counterpoint to any retirement ideology of a life of ease. On the whole, it is consistent with Judeo-Christian thought.

In short, elderly persons as well as others, if they are able to do so, should devote considerable energy to caring for the young and for one another generally. Caring for the young has no priority when an elderly person has competing obligations to others who are old, but when possible, the covenant with the younger generation should be actively fulfilled. Judaism, with its emphasis on the teaching role of the old, and Christianity, with its high valuation of children, can readily encourage this ethic of stewardship by elders for the young.

The Elderly Population and Material Resources

One manifestation of covenantal obligations to the young would be a reluctance to waste scarce resources. Extravagance does not make a mortal immortal. As old persons become more and more numerous in the decades ahead, they should not, for instance, utilize resources in a *futile* struggle against death. Futility, or course, is hard to define; but some elderly persons need to be liberated from the view that death is "wrong," and should develop a reasonable suspicion of the doctrine "Whatever can be done, medically, should be done."

Elderly people need to understand that the value of health competes with other equally important social values, such as education and housing. Medical progress is unlimited, and every step on the path brings new costs. Judeo-Christian thought, while placing considerable trust in individual conscience, also requires social responsibility. An elderly person might well reject some medical interventions that would impoverish his or her children, or that promise very limited benefit at high societal cost. Roman Catholic thought has always maintained that individual choice should be informed by a social conscience committed to the common good, so that "extraordinary" interventions can be refused because of the economic burdens they impose on loved ones (Dedek, 1975). However, this social-mindedness is age-neutral. It is not outlandish to argue that Americans need to lower their expectations of what medicine should promise and what society should provide when it comes to expensive, technology-intensive interventions. However, this argument should not be directed at any particular age group, lest a reasonable proposition for change be immediately dismissed as ageist.

The covenant between generations includes both the wisdom that holds that death is a natural aspect of the life cycle, and the wisdom that holds that duties to the young are important. Unless these duties are fulfilled through service coupled with a rejection of material excess, and through a commitment to justice for all, the circle of reciprocity that defines the intergenerational covenant cannot be sustained.

The old must guard against what theological ethicist William F. May describes as an inclination to "clutch at possessions" that intensifies the "closer one gets to the final dispossession of death" (1982, p. 36). He notes that in the late Middle Ages, avarice was identified as the "chief besetting sin of the aged" by Christian theologians (p. 56). Self-centeredness and avarice, though perhaps understandable responses to mortality, are, in the last analysis, morally inappropriate. In addition, they set a bad example for the young, who naturally look to the old for moral example.

Rationing and the Common Good

Human communities are easily fragmented. The appearance of social harmony often shows itself to be a thin veneer at most. A harmonious and civilized society must remain unambiguously committed to caring for both the young and the old. As Senator Daniel Patrick Moynihan has written: "A commonplace of political rhetoric has it that the quality of a civilization may be measured by how it cares for its elderly. Just as surely, the future of a society may be forecast by how it cares for its young" (1987, p. 194). There is no place for "either . . . or" in this formulation, only for "both . . . and," or justice for all.

Proposals for age-based rationing lead society away from equal human dignity, and reasonable self-determination informed by social conscience, toward a world in which some of the most vulnerable among us become grist in a utilitarian mill. Equality, heterogeneity, self-determination, and social justice need not be mutually exclusive. However much appeal proposals for age-based rationing may have, in the final analysis more is lost than gained through their implementation. Society cannot break its covenant with the older generation and still maintain the common good.

A broken covenant could even lead to mercy killing of elderly individuals. Because such a practice would inevitably be abused, and because it might encourage suicide among elderly persons, it should be resisted (Post, 1990). It is likely that age-based rationing, which condemns the elderly to an otherwise avoidable downward course, would make suicide and mercy killing a more attractive alternative (Battin, 1987). This is a not insignificant reason for the rejection of such rationing proposals. Advocates of age-based rationing demur that their proposals do not in theory entail mercy killing, and they are logically correct. However, the wider public impact of such proposals might be to engender an acceptance of mercy killing as an alternative to the protracted morbidity imposed by age-based cutoffs of heath care.

References

Abernethy, G.L. (1959). *The idea of equality*. Richmond, Va.: John Knox Press.
Augustine (1950). *The city of God*. New York: Modern Library.
Barash, D.P. (1983). *Aging: an exploration*. Seattle: University of Washington Press.

Battin, M.P. (1987). Age rationing and the just distribution of health care: is there a duty to die? In T.M. Smeeding, ed., *Should medical care be rationed by age?*, pp. 69–94. Totowa, N.J.: Rowman & Littlefield.

Berdyaev, N. (1957). *Dostoevsky.* New York: Meridian.

Bernardin, J. (1985). Health care and the consistent ethic of life. *Origins, 15*(3), 36–40.

Butler, R.N. (1975). *Why survive? being old in America.* New York: Harper and Row.

Cadoux, C.J. (1925). *The early church and the world.* Edinburgh: T. & T. Clark.

Callahan, D. (1987). *Setting limits: medical goals in an aging society.* New York: Simon & Schuster.

Callahan, D. (1990). *What kind of life: the limits of medical progress.* New York: Simon & Schuster.

Cassirer, E. (1944). *An essay on man.* New Haven: Yale University Press.

Childress, J.F. (1982). *Who should decide? paternalism in healthcare.* New York: Oxford University Press.

Childress, J.F. (1984). Ensuring care, respect, and fairness for the elderly. *Hastings Center Report, 14*(5), 27–31.

Crystal, S. (1982). *America's old age crisis: the two worlds of aging.* New York: Basic Books.

Dedek, J.F. (19795). *Contemporary medical ethics.* Kansas City: Sheed, Andrews, & McMeel.

Durkheim, E. (1965). *The elementary forms of religious life.* New York: Free Press.

Feldman, D.M. (1986). *Health and medicine in the Jewish tradition.* New York: Crossroad.

Fletcher, J. (1988). Ethics and old age. *Update: Ethics Center of Loma Linda University, 4*(1), 2–5.

Gallop, G. (1981). *Gallop Opinion Index: religion in America.* Princeton, N.J.: American Institute of Public Opinion.

Green, R.M. (1988). *Religion and moral reason: a new method for comparative study.* New York: Oxford University Press.

Herzog, A.R., Holden, K., and Seltzer, M. (1989). *Older women: research issues and data sources.* Amityville, N.Y.: Baywood.

Herschel, A. (1959). *Between God and man: an interpretation of Judaism.* New York: Free Press.

Kant, I. (1964). *Groundwork of the metaphysics of morals*, translated by H.J. Patton. New York: Harper & Row.

Kass, L.R. (1985). *Toward a more natural science: biology and human affairs.* New York: Free Press.

Kilner, J.F. (1984). Who shall be saved? an African answer. *Hastings Center Report, 14*(3), 18–22.

Lopata, H.Z., ed. (1987). *Widows*, 2 vols. Durham, N.C.: Duke University Press.

May, W.F. (1982). Who cares for the elderly? *Hastings Center Report, 12*(6), 31–37.

Motokiyo, Z. (1977). The deserted crone. In G.L. Anderson, ed., *Masterpieces of the Orient*, pp. 712–720. New York: W.W. Norton & Co.

Moynihan, D. (1987). *Family and nation*. New York: Harcourt Brace Jovanovich.

Nouwen, H., and Gaffney, W. (1974). *Aging: the fulfillment of life*. Garden City, N.Y.: Doubleday.

Post, S.G. (1990). Severely demented elderly people: the case against senecide. *Journal of the American Geriatrics Society, 38*, 715–718.

Preston, S.H. (1984). Children and the elderly in the U.S. *Scientific American, 251*(6), 44–49.

Protzman, F. (1989). Killing of 49 elderly patients by nurse aides stuns Austria. *New York Times*, April 18, p. 1.

Riley, M.W., and Riley, J.W., Jr. (1986). Longevity and social structure: the potential of added years. In L. Bronte and A. Pifer, eds., *Our aging society: paradox and promise*, pp. 53–77. New York: W.W. Norton & Co.

Sapp, S. (1987). *Full of years: aging and the elderly in the bible and today*, Nashville, Tenn.: Abingdon.

Simmons, L.W. (1945). *The role of the aged in primitive society*. New Haven, Conn.: Yale University Press.

Staniforth, M., ed. (1968). *Early Christian writings: the apostolic fathers*. New York: Penguin.

Walzer, M. (1985). *Exodus and revolution*. New York: Basic Books.

Zaner, R.M. (1988). *Ethics and the clinical encounter*. Englewood Cliffs, N.J.: Prentice Hall.

7

From Ageism toward Autonomy

DAVID C. THOMASMA, Ph.D.

"You tell him he's unnecessary and that is a . . . sin . . . It's abortion at the other end."
—*Nat in "I'm Not Rappaport," by Herb Gardner*

As Larry Churchill has suggested, to set limits to health care is inimical to the American spirit. Our vision of rugged individualism and limitless frontiers to conquer, our crusades of mercy and wars on poverty, and our social commitments despite a capricious form of social justice are all examples of that spirit.

Nowhere is the idea of setting limits more repugnant than when considering health care for elderly Americans (Churchill, 1987, p. 20). Caring for the elderly plays an important role in our social vision of the kind of society we want to be. This deeper vision can be detected in our original legislative goals for caring for the elderly.

However, these legislative goals, and the vision that animated them, have largely vanished. In their place is increasing social pressure for limiting access to health care on the basis of age. The social contract itself may have to change precisely because of the aging of the citizenry (Madigan, 1989).

This chapter sets forth an argument against such ageism on philosophical grounds, where *ageism* stands for the use of an age cutoff in allocating scarce medical resources. Nonetheless, philosophical argumentation alone is insufficient to properly address ageism and must be complemented by the range of analysis represented in this volume.

This chapter will present a number of ageist proposals for resolving the problem of limited resources in health care, followed by a critique of these proposals, largely on the basis of their internal consistency. Next, it will develop the importance of paying attention to individuals' wishes in constructing a system for resource allocation. Last, it will propose a social program that requires that advance directives be obtained. The conclusion emphasizes that self-determination should be taken into account in health care policy.

Ageist Proposals

As continued gerification—continued increased overall aging—takes hold in society, our cherished values are placed increasingly at risk. We cannot currently resolve our problems in dealing with the aged. How will it be possible to do so when so many more people become dependent on the rest of us for care, compassion, support, time, energy, and resources? Fifty years from now, it is projected, nearly one-quarter of the population will be aged 65 and older, and more than 12 million persons will be over age 85 (U.S. Senate, Special Committee on Aging, 1989).

Pressures for Rationing

Unbearable social burdens are projected to occur as a result of improved longevity. In part, this longevity is a result of greater control of infection in hospitals and in society. However, it is also due to an enormous number of life-prolonging and life-sustaining technologies. Among them are resuscitation, ventilator support, body-part replacements, antibiotics, dialysis, and nutritional support and hydration (U.S. Congress, Office of Technology Assessment, 1987). Americans want the very best care for everyone without restrictions, but they are generally unwilling to pay for any costs in excess of the current expenditures. As technology expands, rationing seems inevitable (Kapp, 1989a).

The two major problems caused by increased longevity, then, are increased cost and human choice. As successive reports claim that the costs of health care will continue to increase in the 1990s, greater and greater attention has been focused on limiting those costs by limiting individuals' access to health care. As the U.S. Congress, Office of Technology Assessment puts it:

> Concurrently, rising health care costs and expenditures have generated widespread public concern and have led to changes in medical practices in private insurance and public programs that pay for medical care—changes intended to limit health care costs and spending. The pressure for cost containment has added another dimension to the debate about life-sustaining technologies. (1987, p. 39)

The technologies themselves also require human choices about their application and appropriateness, as well as about their withdrawal and inappropriateness. The use of technologies that cannot cure but can only ameliorate are the bane of current health care programs. In this context, the cost of chronic care, especially in nursing homes, is beginning to exceed our society's ability to pay for it (Jennings et al., 1988; also see chapter 2, above). The right to live and to die is inexorably bound to medical technology and its use in the care of elderly patients.

Learning to say no to dramatic, life-prolonging technology is an important part of providing for the future (Boyle, 1984; Thurow, 1984), but at present the nay-saying seems focused on society's limiting access to resources rather than on enabling individuals to make their own choice. The freedom of elderly persons in this context (Thomasma, 1984) and in the context of long-term care (Hofland, 1988) is fundamentally compromised. New efforts to foster the autonomy of the elderly are needed.

Efforts to control technology and human choice must be carried out in an atmosphere of growing concern about the political power of elderly Americans. Are they now taking a greater share of the goods and resources of society than is their due? If so, will this trend continue, such that—as described in the opening chapter of this book—a social backlash will add to the pressure for limiting health care for the elderly that the Office of Technology Assessment (1987) describes? These concerns force everyone to take ageist proposals seriously. Such proposals are based on hard realities.

Many persons agree that some solution to the problem of access to health care needs to be found as our populace ages (Callahan, 1987a; Daniels, 1985; Daniels, 1988; President's Commission, 1983). However, allocating access to health care on the basis of age or other demographic criteria violates the inherent ethical principles of medicine and of health care, and, for that matter, the principles of justice in society. But what alternatives are there?

The rationing of health care resources certainly must be considered, but not on ageist grounds. How can it be done ethically? Increased squeezing of the health care dollar through social policies such as DRGs (diagnosis-related groups) and a freeze on Medicare fees, as well as the inability of some states to honor Medicaid bills submitted by hospitals and nursing homes, have created a tremendous crisis in the health care system. At root is the loss of personal and professional control over decisions. This control is now lodged in a bureaucracy that is itself so expensive that some physicians suggest abolishing it to save money.

This sentiment in favor of abolishing the health care bureaucracy is echoed by many, and in increasing numbers. Thirty-seven million Americans cannot get access to health care because they have no health insurance; one-third of them are children. Medicaid serves a decreasing proportion of the poor, no more than two-fifths altogether, and our infant mortality rate is among the highest in the developed world (Cohn,

1989). Charges of institutional racism in the health care system have been made, along with charges of human rights violations in the failure to provide life-extending medical care to persons who are dying (*Medical Ethics Advisor*, 1989d).

A poll of Americans, published in 1989, indicated that 90 percent wanted key changes in health care. Canadians and Britishers were also polled, and only about 1 percent indicated that they would exchange their national health plans for the American system. Since Americans have a worse survival rate at birth and a shorter life expectancy than the Canadians and the Britishers, this does not come as a surprise (Millenson, 1989). When Margaret Thatcher offered a plan for the first overhaul of the British system by introducing more competition, she was roundly criticized, even by doctors, who vowed to fight the changes (though they had once vowed to fight the National Health Service itself, not unlike the American Medical Association, which fights any changes in our own system). Although overburdened, the health service was called "poor" only by 15 percent of the Britishers polled. As one observer said about Thatcher's plan, it might "prove the first step on the road to the horror of the American health system" (Longworth, 1989, p. 10).

When such astounding numbers of uninsured Americans cannot get access to health care, many observers think that "some form of universal health care" is "inevitable." These same proponents can point to surveys that show "consistent support for a tax-supported egalitarian national program" (Hope and Young, 1988, p. 23). Mainstream groups, such as Consumers Union, criticize the current system and argue that consumers cannot look to the private sector to finance and support long-term care, and therefore must look to government (*Chicago Tribune*, 1989). As Harry Moody (1988) has argued, however, our government has been most successful in shifting difficult and sensitive allocation issues to the private sector, professionals, and even the court system.

There is considerable concern about a universal health care plan, which would also "inevitably" impose rationing by means of first-come-first-served policies that might back up elective surgery, for example, for almost six months (*Hospitals*, 1988; Weinstein, 1988). Major efforts will have to be made to strengthen cooperation so as to control technology in the patchwork system that now exists (Franklin, 1988). Among the more creative plans are those that emphasize more local and personal control over allocation decisions (Beck, 1989); however, such control should not be used by the government as an excuse for not making hard decisions. A good example of such a plan might be a systematic process developed by both patients and physicians, using the hospital ethics committee itself (La Puma et al., 1988). As Carola Eisenberg, a physician, emphasizes, "We must mobilize our natural allies—our patients and the public at large. It is they who have the greatest stake in the battle to preserve excellence in medical care" (Eisenberg, 1986, p. 1113). It is within this context that discussions about access to health care for aged Americans should be held.

Proposals for Rationing

The first proposal to be considered here is that of former Governor Lamm of Colorado. When he presented a major address "The Ten Commandments of an Aging Society," a few years ago, his ninth commandment was "Do not let young children suffer because of health care we give the elderly" (Lamm, 1987). In fact, all he proposes is that spending on the elderly be curtailed on the basis of a utilitarian social policy. Lamm says that, in order to obtain the greatest good for the greatest number, funds must be left over from health care to provide for other social needs. Because of the increasing gerification of society, cutoffs must be made. Since the greatest good also requires that other social goods go to the workers who both provide for the future and provide the care for the elderly, and to the children who will be the workers of the future, ageist criteria should be employed (Lamm, 1985, pp. 35–50).

Lamm is critical of what he calls "antisocial ethics." This is an ethics of emotional appeal, which exhorts society to care for the elderly. While sounding exalted, it actually hurts society. In his view, "it is an irresponsible allocation of resources to finance machines and techniques which drain our pocketbooks but yield limited results." He also decries "media-driven humanity," by which he means individual appeals for resources sponsored by the media while thousands of unpublicized patients go untreated (Hafka, 1985).

Since two-thirds of the cost of providing health care for elderly Americans is borne by the government by means of Medicare and Medicaid, it is not surprising that Lamm, as an elected official, targeted the aged population in his proposals. A second consideration is that by comparison with other members of society, elderly persons use a disproportionate share (in Lamm's view) of health care costs. Thus, limits on their care would have more immediately noticeable effects in terms of utilitarian policy than would cutoffs imposed on other groups (Kapp, 1989a, p. 5).

A second, less rigid proposal is that made by Daniel Callahan, whose concerns are like Lamm's. Callahan's proposal is based on the concept of a natural lifespan. The government would be required to help persons live out a natural lifespan, with attention to quality of life. After that time, perhaps when the individual reaches age 80 or so, the use of expensive medical technology would not be allowed (Callahan, 1987a; Callahan 1987b).

Callahan's proposal has considerable merit. In it, the elderly are encouraged to sacrifice their access to life-extending technological resources in favor of future generations, while simultaneously being supported by society in terms of guarantees for their own quality of life. Callahan avoids the fallacy of equating access to sophisticated technology with good-quality care. He correctly sees that the high cost of care is created by the ever-increasing development of sophisticated medical technology and the growing numbers of patients admitted to technology-intensive institutions (Callahan, 1986). Thus, his is a more sophisticated understanding of the balance between care and support by society than is found in other proposals. As he sees it, rationing by categorical standards (such as age, outcome assessment, and cost) is far superior to leaving the decision to a case-by-case assessment at the bedside (Callahan, 1989).

In his most recent work, Callahan tackles the difficult question of what society will consider to be sufficient health care, offering principles for judging such sufficiency (1990, pp. 123–134). One principle is that "an absence of good health does not account for a deficiency in the functioning of its [society's] major social institutions" (p. 127). Another is the principle of full accounting, according to which resources must not be harmfully diverted form other needs (p. 131). Callahan also proposes various levels of care that can be effectively used for public policy purposes (pp. 176–177). These "curative priorities" help flesh out but do not fundamentally alter his central thesis.

Further, Callahan argues for a more balanced notion of the community than is found in utilitarian accounts. He emphasizes human interconnectedness and continuity. Under his plan, elderly persons would be encouraged to be selfless rather than to insist on individual entitlements. The limitations in health care would therefore focus on acute medical treatment that is primarily oriented toward life prolongation but has not been proven to enhance the quality of life. Interventions that are oriented toward providing comfort, relieving suffering, and improving mental and physical functioning would continue.

A third view is that of Norman Daniels, who argues that a prospective national policy, in which citizens decide ahead of time that certain technologies would be ruled out for all persons beyond a specified age, would be a just method of allocating resources (Daniels, 1985; Daniels, 1988). This is called a prudential plan model, since each person would, knowing ahead of time what to expect, prudently plan for the future. Daniels's model relies upon a "veil of ignorance," a method of thinking derived from philosopher John Rawls. If everyone were "ig-

norant" about both their future health and economic status, then prudent deliberators would opt for a scheme that would improve their
chances of reaching a normal lifespan, in preference to one that would
reduce their chances of reaching a normal lifespan but improve their
chances of further longevity once a normal lifespan had been achieved.

Daniels provides a definition of intergenerational justice that is very
important. Intergenerational obligations would entail that each generation be provided with what is needed to have an equal opportunity to
compete for goods and services to reach the next developmental stage
of life. Because all persons are growing older, there is no discrimination
if all persons together know ahead of time that certain goods and
services will be cut off at an advanced age. He has concluded that "there
are conditions under which a health-care system that rationed life-
extending resources by age would be the prudent choice and therefore
the choice that constituted a just or fair distribution of resources between
age groups" (Daniels, 1988, p. 91). Nor is such a scheme a violation
of equality. Unlike sexism and racism, differential treatment by age is
not incompatible with treating people equally. As Daniels notes, "If we
treat the young one way and the old another, then over time, each
person is treated both ways. The advantages (or disadvantages) of consistent differential treatment by age equalizes over time" (Daniels, as
quoted in Kilner, 1988, p. 405).

According to a fourth proposal, by Robert Veatch, health care
rationing could be done along egalitarian lines. According to such a
scheme, persons would receive "priority claims" to health care resources
in inverse proportion to their chronological age. That is, younger persons would have a higher priority than would older ones for access to
certain life-prolonging technology. Rationing would be done not on the
basis of age but rather on the basis of priorities. (However, these priorities seem only to thinly mask age-based rationing.) As individuals age,
they have already used some of their social power to compete for goods
and services and have less claim than others on future resources (Veatch,
1988). Although Veatch says that he is opposed to rationing on the
basis of age, this model still uses age as a criterion for determining
access to the goods and services of society.

All four of the proposals discussed above, as well as others that
have been made (see Smeeding, 1987), would use age as a criterion for
withholding care, but they represent quite different approaches. It would
be inappropriate to think negatively of them solely on the basis of "gut
reactions" against age-based discrimination. They raise important points
that ought to be absorbed into any comprehensive program for the care
of elderly Americans.

When the particular positions of each thinker are abstracted, the following five principles emerge:

* The rationing of health care is needed.
* Such rationing should focus on modes of care that are expensive and less effective, rather than on expensive but effective care.
* Even though rationing will occur, it should not impede social support for elderly Americans or lower their quality of life.
* All citizens should know ahead of time what categories of care will and will not be provided in the different stages of their lifespan.
* Any social policy should foster intergenerational justice and altruism.

A Critique of Ageism

Despite the important values noted above, the problems with these proposals are enormous. First, even with the best-laid plans, individuals often are not responsible for illnesses they contract, especially later in life. Thus, individuals must be treated in an individual manner. This is the strength of Daniels's proposal, and a weakness of both Lamm's and Callahan's. While it certainly seems reasonable to curtail spending on technology-intensive medical care, most of the spending done by elderly persons and their families is for nursing home care and chronic care, something even Callahan would not deny for the elderly. Hence his proposal is criticized because it will not save money in the long run.

Furthermore, the concept of a "natural life-span" is hard to defend in a society so well developed as ours. What are we to do with the many patients over age 80 or 85? People undergo surgery when they are over 100 years of age, and do well. There are many studies, such as the Baltimore Longitudinal Study of Aging (Shock et al., 1984) and the work done by Fries and Crapo (1981), that demonstrate rather clearly that physiologic age correlates poorly with chronological age. Age itself is a very poor criterion for judging who should and who should not receive life-prolonging technology (Fries and Crapo, 1981; Shock et al., 1984). While we can admit with Callahan that a person's age is part of his or her own self-understanding, and influences society's behavior toward that person (Callahan, 1987b), age itself does not qualify as the best criterion to use in allocating assistance to individuals who wish to survive.

There is a fundamental inconsistency in Callahan's thesis. If we are to cut off technology-intensive care, as Callahan and others propose, surely it is doubly cruel for such thinkers to close their minds to steps that would end suffering, such as withdrawing food and water from patients at their request (Callahan, 1983), or even voluntary, active euthanasia (Thomasma, 1988b). Both euthanasia and assisted suicide are seen by Callahan as being disrespectful of elderly persons. Yet, ironically, given his concerns about cost containment, these activities would surely cut down on the aggregate expenses of dying. Approximately 30 percent of the total costs of Medicare and Medicaid are incurred by patients who are in their last 12 months of life. Admittedly, values other than cost containment must also be protected in any scheme for allocating health care. It is right for Callahan to protect the intrinsic value of human life; but once external factors, such as the social welfare of all, economics, or a national health policy that limits treatment on the basis of a natural lifespan, are used to allocate care, the intrinsic value of the individual is at risk.

The basic reason to oppose treating elderly Americans differently than other citizens, however, is one of social commitment. What sort of society ought we to be? Should we not treat all forms of human life equally? If we do not, and have no objective standards (leaving judgments instead to be formed on subjective, quality-of-life standards), then how can we avoid becoming a much poorer form of political society than we are today (Thomasma, 1989b)? After all, the principle of intergenerational justice cuts both ways. If, as Callahan proposes, elderly persons must be encouraged to sacrifice for the young, why cannot young persons be urged to sacrifice for the elderly? It is the latter group that has "sacrificed" throughout life, building a family, working, helping directly or indirectly through taxes to develop the roads, the bridges, the symphonies and schools, the parks and the businesses, that make up the enormous range of social goods and services the young now enjoy. In particular, as Abrams noted, what kind of justice is it that deprives elderly citizens of the results of medical research when their taxes financed the discoveries (Hafka, 1985)?

In this respect, one could argue against Daniels's thesis that prudential deliberators would choose a system of equality behind the veil of ignorance. What if, instead, they would choose one that honors the elderly more than it does the young, as many other societies in the world do today? This would be a nonegalitarian model of intergenerational justice. Consider a practical example. As Kapp points out, the Medicare Catastrophic Coverage Act of 1988 was the first example of social policy that explicitly rested on the principle of "generational equity" (Kapp, 1989b, p. 6). According to this principle, every group, ideally every individual, with the exception of the very young, would support himself or herself without subsidies from other groups (Longman, 1987). Considering the reaction to the Catastrophic Coverage Act, the elderly themselves would certainly not opt for the principle of generational equity if they were included among the prudential deliberators! In fact, many of the rest of us would object to this principle on the grounds that it betrays too individualistic and unsympathetic a view of human society and interconnectedness. The elderly are our parents and grandparents; and a person may be loved and cherished by others throughout his or her life-span.

Finally, when looked at closely, many thinkers who seem to propose age as a criterion for access to certain forms of care are seen to actually employ age as a shorthand for more complicated social concepts (Thomasma, 1988a). These concepts include competition for the goods and services of society, intergenerational justice, and the like. Age is also used as a shorthand for features clinically relevant to allocation, such as weakness or debilitation. Joseph Fletcher contends that research into longevity and advances in medical practice will lead to the existence of senescent beings in young bodies, since brain cells themselves do not regenerate. This insight, and not the specific age of a person, should be the driving force for allocation decisions. Even though individual ethics should be developed within the context of social morality, Fletcher argues that individual lives should end not by social imposition (as seems to be the case with ageism) but by individual choice, when the individual no longer perceives an adequate quality of life (Fletcher, 1988).

A Basic Right to Health Care

A right to health care for all citizens must be developed and implemented, but it would have to exist within a context of overall rationing. Such a context is important. As Scitovsky and Capron (1986) have shown, health care costs are at least partially driven by the practice of "doing everything possible" for patients due to a lack of clear social guidelines and to fear of liability. A typical clinical reaction to rationing is offered by Robert Scheer, a physician: "In the absence of a clearly stated instruction from the patient, I cannot stop artificial kidney treatments, regardless of how useless such treatments may have become in saving the patient's life" (1985, p. 26). As Albert Jonsen points out, however, life must be supported by love; the personal perception of one's history; and by engagement, "however simple, in the ongoing currents of the social and natural world. Unless our life-support technology can support such life, it is empty of human significance" (1988, p. 68).

The components of an argument for a basic right to health care might be the following:

Experience

The experience of a well-designed social system in which all persons have access to health care can easily be gained by consulting Canadian, British, and other European models. Americans may be embarrassed by our nation's lack of resolution of the problem of access, especially when confronted by European colleagues. Uwe Reinhardt, a medical economist at Princeton University who is familiar with different models from different countries, has very clearly laid out the strengths and weaknesses of the American system of access to health care as compared to the European (Reinhardt, 1986). Its strength is its freedom; its weaknesses are apparent in its lack of compassion and of justice.

Data and Demographics

We are unable (read, unwilling) to provide access to health care for almost 37 million under- and uninsured Americans. These people are not all abjectly poor; some work for companies without health insurance policies, or have temporarily lost their jobs. The poor have had their access to medical care restricted by hospital closings in inner cities or rural areas, such that obtaining care, while still possible (perhaps at a county hospital) has become less and less convenient (Franklin, 1989). Because we cannot now address the needs of our citizens major unmet needs—unless there is a drastic change in the near future, a social revolutionary kind of change—will rupture our society. For this reason, support for some sort of national health insurance like that discussed by the Physicians for a National Health Plan is required. What might emerge would be a multitiered social program like the one I call "eldercare," rather than a program in which the federal government is the sole insurer. In any case, the disparity created by uneven access is a violation of the general principles of justice, and a violation of the principle of treating each person as if he or she were a class instance of the human race (Pellegrino and Thomasma, 1981).

Philosophical Reasoning

A social decision is required to define Americans' fundamental rights to health care (Pellegrino and Thomasma, 1981, p. 278). As MacIntyre has so persuasively argued, practical rationality must be part and parcel of a particular social setting, such as medical care, and that particular social setting may not conform to abstract, general conceptions of justice. Moreover, as he notes, disagreement and conflict are endemic to any such setting.

We not only move away from theories according to which the exercise of practical rationality presupposes some kind of social setting, but we move into a world in which the exercise of practical rationality, if it is to occur at all, has to be embodied in social contexts of fundamental disagreement and conflict. (MacIntyre, 1988, p. 325)

A good example of disagreement and conflict arises when we consider certain libertarian notions of practical rationality. Some of us might be appalled by the reasoning of libertarians such as Nozick, Engelhardt, and recently Rie. The latter two authors published an article that proposed skimming and dumping (getting the paying patients, and dumping off those who can't pay on the public system) as "virtues," since private-enterprise hospitals then teach society to make its own commitments to the poor (Engelhardt and Rie, 1988). The libertarian view of society is essentially flawed because it is based on a social-contract theory that emphasizes autonomy as a condition of possibility for ethics (Engelhardt, 1987). In this view, the fact that some persons cannot get access to health care is unfortunate but not unjust. No one has a claim on the resources of others unless by social and explicit contact.

This is not the kind of society we ought to be. The issues of the right to health care are to be played out in conflicting views of the nature of human society, whether they be libertarian or egalitarian, or based on the bonds of compassion (Loewy, 1989). Respect for autonomy is important, but beneficence-in-trust is the primary ethical principle, not respect for autonomy (which is included in the principle). This principle governs especially the relationships of need and meeting needs that occur in health care (Pellegrino and Thomasma, 1988).

If we ration health care on the basis of age, serious difficulties arise for justice and for the nature of our society. Among those difficulties are inequities of access, a lack of respect for aged persons in spite of all they have done for the younger generations, the creation of institutional dumping grounds for incompetent persons and the elderly, and the withholding of care from many elderly individuals who could profit from it and return to a normal life.

Is there some way to avoid the ageist social policies discussed above? Can there be a sophisticated and complex policy that would empower individuals in a grassroots movement for medical ethics and social policy (Carwile, 1988)?

Autonomy and Elderly People

The reason that argumentation alone cannot confront the power of ageist proposals is that nothing short of a "social revolution" will be able to address the health care needs of the massive numbers of elderly persons who will need some support in the future. Recall the demographics. Within 50 years, the number of dependent persons will increase almost tenfold.

I use the term *social revolution* because the necessary changes will require rethinking of the freedoms we normally assign to one another. The scope of this chapter does not allow for the development of the components of the entire program. Instead, I will focus on the role of self-determination in a major social policy designed to care for elderly Americans. The primary point is to underscore ways in which individuals might gain more control over expensive medical technology. While aiding themselves and their values, they would also assist society in controlling costs and would lessen, but not eliminate, the impact of rationing.

Medical ethics differ in one significant respect from the traditional humanities. The latter deal with real and imagined persons and events, seen through the lens of time; but in medical ethics there is an immediacy that is both poignant and challenging. That is why it appeals to so many people. Each person has a story from his or her own life that relates directly to the issues discussed in medical ethics. Invariably when more theoretical considerations are discussed in medical ethics, participants will relate these to concrete persons and events in their own life. There is no need to reconstruct how Greece or Rome or the Middle Ages viewed duties towards persons: This is now. This is my grandfather. This is my grandmother. This is the nursing home. That is the feeding tube. This is the loss of independence. That is the stroke.

Little can be gained by assuming simplistic postures about any one of the incredibly complex issues that do arise when technology meets human life. However, there does seem to be a difference between the issues that arise at the beginning of life and those that arise at the end of life: between obstetric and pediatric issues, and geriatric ones. In the former instances we may sometimes be dealing with potential human beings. Although such beings have rights, they may be more restricted than those of fully functioning human beings. Thus, a frozen embryo might, in the future, acquire the right to be implanted (as it apparently now has in Australia), but not, of course, the rights of free speech, assembly, suffrage, and the like, which we honor in adult persons (those who are able to make moral choices). At the end of life, we are dealing with persons who have constructed a value history. Even if a few pediatric patients and a few geriatric patients are now both considered incompetent, there is a world of difference between them.

The heart of the difference lies in the fulfillment of the capacity to make decisions on the basis of either the values individuals already have or the values that emerge after reflection on the options. Although all beings should be valued by us, and their integrity should be preserved as far as possible when a tragic choice is forced on us, it is far easier to decide about applying a medical technology or withholding it altogether on the basis of the values constructed by a patient over a lifetime than on the basis of a "valueless" field presented by the embryo or the newborn. At least in theory, debates about the living will and other means of controlling the application of medical technologies at the end of life should be less intense than those about abortion and the care of defective newborns (Mauro, 1988). Honoring the individual patient's values by incorporating them into the decisions to be made about that patient, once he or she becomes incompetent, is the primary way we can respect patients' inherent dignity. If they are dying, we should never strip them of the lifetime of choices their values represent.

A position of solid commitment to the value of human life, even when the life in question may no longer belong to a human person as we normally understand personhood, produces the safest insurance against bigotry, repression, neo-Nazism, and murder. This position becomes a truism if there is no attempt to define the kinds of efforts that will be required in directing technology. Some important examples are worth discussing.

Controlling the use of life-prolonging technologies is but one aspect of the larger problem of applying technology to human aims. Nowhere is this more apparent than in the application of medical technology and its various interventions to the aged and dying patient. There is a fallacy in thinking that everyone wants "the very best" medical technology. The fallacy involved equates advanced technology with better care. Not surprisingly, studies have confirmed that it is not the technology but the care a person receives that determines his or her well-being and, in the case of the elderly patient, the protection of his or her human spirit to the end (Chicago Tribune, 1986).

Dramatic changes in health care have also resulted in a movement away from the more personal and familial types of care. There has been an enormous increase in the technologization of care. Where once a cold compress might have been applied and the patient's hand held, now all sorts of interventions are possible, from the use of intravenous fluids and nutrition, blood products and agents to prevent clotting or bleeding, and cardiopulmonary resuscitation, to the use of experimental treatments such as advanced chemotherapeutic agents, radiologic implants, artificial hearts, and transplantation of various organs. For the most part, these interventions are much better than a cold compress! However, to the extent that personal control over the dying process is lost, new protections must be developed.

Personal control of the aging process (and later, the dying process) can be regained by appealing to a number of the principles of medical ethics. Some of these have now been recognized in the law as well. One obvious one is that of informed consent. This standard originally was applied to medical research, but in *Canterbury v. Spence* (1972) it was applied by the District of Columbia Circuit Court to customary medical treatment. According to this principle, individuals have a right to decide about their own medical treatment, and must be given sufficient information and freedom to make that choice. As Russell McIntyre (1988) notes about a New Jersey Supreme Court adoption of the "objective prudent patient standard" in regard to informed consent, the obligation of providing information and being sure the patient is free to make the decision falls on the physician, and the requirement to pursue this obligation is linked, in New Jersey at least, to other New Jersey Supreme Court judgments regarding the right to die. These other judgments involve protection of the rights of patients.

All adult patients should have a right to refuse treatment, even if this refusal might lead to their death. Court cases, such as *In re Bartling* (1984, 1986) in California, and *In re Conroy* (1985) and *In re Jobes* (1986) in New Jersey, have confirmed this right, even for incompetent patients. An incompetent patient does not lose the right to refuse treatment; a guardian or a family member must speak for his or her wishes. Thus, the family does not have a right to say what it would want, so much as what the patient would prefer. This right is sustained by the U.S. Constitution whether or not there is living-will legislation in a given patient's state. Of course, a living will strengthens the advance directive a patient gives about his or her care. Perhaps the strongest statement comes from California in the case of Elizabeth Bouvia. There the California Second District Court of Appeals stated explicitly that a patient has the right to refuse any medical treatment and that the exercise of this right requires no one's approval (*Ethical Currents*, 1986).

However, in what was characterized as a setback for the right-to-die movement, the Missouri Supreme Court forbade the withdrawal of artificial nutrition and hydration through a gastrostomy in the case of Nancy Cruzan, who had lain in a permanent vegetative state for 5 years as a result of an automobile accident. She was then 30 years old. If the feeding continues, she might be expected to live another 30 years in this condition. Her family had argued that she did not wish to live in this condition. Their argument was based on a somewhat serious conversation in which Nancy had indicated that if sick or injured she would not want to have her life continued unless she could live "halfway normally." A trial court found this sufficient evidence that she would not want to live maintained only on artificial food and hydration, and ordered the state employees caring for her in the Mount Vernon State Hospital to carry out the request of her legal guardians to withdraw the fluids and nutrition.

On appeal, however, the Missouri Supreme Court brushed aside the nearly 100 court cases in 20 states, and the living-will statutes in 38 states including Missouri itself (*Cruzan v. Harmon*, 1988). The overwhelming majority of the court cases had been decided in favor of the right to die (Society for the Right to Die, 1989). These cases also affirmed the role of families or other decision makers who are able to say, in the absence of written statements from patients, that the patient would not have wanted the treatments in question (p. 2). The statutes are based on the right of individuals to determine their own treatment, especially when they are dying.

In the Cruzan case, the Missouri Supreme Court considered that euphemisms were given undue prominence in the cases they looked to for precedent, particularly the concept that if fluids and nutrition were withdrawn, the patient would die of the underlying disease. The majority opinion (4 to 3) held that the constitutional right to privacy is not expansive enough to apply to life-saving treatment. Other court decisions, different from the Missouri one, were simply based on a desire to interpret the law in favor of the individual's right to die. Only the United States Supreme Court could make the final interpretation of the constitutional right to privacy (*Medical Ethics Advisor*, 1989b; *Medical Ethics Advisor*, 1989c).

The Missouri decision demonstrates that one can interpret the law in many ways (*Medical Ethics Advisor*, 1989b). Richard McCormick says of the Missouri court's decision on Cruzan that it is, "in my judgment, so bad that it may prove to be pedagogically useful. It is muddled, confused and/or downright wrong on virtually every key issue" (1989, p. 3). Patients who express their wishes about their deaths ahead of time must be respected, if they and their lives are not to be denuded of their values at the end (Thomasma, 1983).

At risk, too, and not very well examined, is the right of the family to advocate and interpret the preferences of their loved ones who become incompetent. In California, a measure by the legislature to broaden the situations under which a living will may apply (usually it only covers the final days of a person's dying process) was vetoed by the governor, apparently in concern that it might excessively relax the definition of death, making it easier for doctors to remove life-sustaining technology

(Coleman, 1989). But that is the whole point! Controlling technology by shaping its use in response to an individual's values is the struggle of this and the next century. As McCormick says further, "human persons have an enormous stake in the quality of their lives—how they live, how they die, and how they live while dying" (1989, p. 3).

One problem in the Missouri case was with the specificity of the patient's wishes. In this regard, the court built upon an earlier and less restrictive judgment handed down in New York regarding Mary O'Connor. The decision in New York is considered less restrictive because it did not deny that patients have the right to express their wishes in the form of advance directives, or that the family might have a legitimate role in witnessing those directives. Rather, it points out that O'Connor did not make any specific spoken reference to or leave any written instructions regarding fluids and nutrition.

She was 77, a widow, with two daughters who were practical nurses. During her later years, she frequently had to confront issues of life prolongation with relatives and with her husband. The daughters and friends were able to testify to her constant and explicit desire never to "be a burden to anyone" and "not to lose [her] dignity"; and to her feeling that it was "monstrous" to keep someone alive using machinery when they are "not going to get any better." She held that people who were suffering very badly should be allowed to die. Several times she told Helen, one of her daughters, that if she became ill and could not take care of herself, she would not want her life to be sustained artificially (*Medical Ethics Advisor*, 1989a). A trial court approved the discontinuation of fluids and nutrition after her progressive deterioration after a series of strokes. She was in a geriatric care center at the time. The appellate court affirmed that ruling, but when the nursing home went to the New York Court of Appeals, the court issued a surprise ruling. After affirming that the ideal situation was to have advance directives from the patient herself, or a living will (which is not yet legal in New York), as well as acknowledging that repeated oral expressions are important, the court overturned the rulings of the lower courts because it was not clear how the patient's statements, as expressed by family and friends, applied to the withdrawal of fluids and nutrition (p. 15).

The Society for the Right to Die commented on this case with respect to the role of the family, as follows:

> the underlying assumption is that to permit ending treatment without clear and convincing evidence would lead to abuse of the vulnerable elderly. Other courts and authorities ... have strongly held that decision-making when the patient is incompetent is best discharged by family members

who know and care for the patient, rather than health care provider or courts, to whom she may be a stranger. (*Medical Ethics Advisor*, 1989a, pp. 15–16)

The court's position is that there is nothing more than conjecture about whether O'Connor would have wanted the fluids and nutrition withdrawn. One suspects, however, that a deeper concern about many vulnerable individuals has now surfaced. This concern has as its deep background the Nazi experience. However, the question remains, how specific can or must individuals be about future contingencies involving their health? It seems sufficient to take seriously the "family principle": that lacking any other data about malicious intent or dysfunction, families should be considered the best interpreters of their loved one's wishes, unless, of course, the family itself is judged incompetent to speak for their loved one for one reason or another (Pellegrino and Thomasma, 1988, pp. 162–171).

The U.S. Supreme Court did make a decision in the Cruzan case that underscores some of these issues. First, it emphasized that a competent patient has the right to refuse all medical treatment, even if such a person is not dying. Second, fluids and nutrition (medically delivered food and water) are to be considered medical treatment, and fall under this right. Third, an incompetent person does not lose the right to refuse treatment, but his or her wishes must be expressed by legally recognized instruments. While the Supreme Court did not say that Nancy Cruzan's parents or surrogates in general could not be considered such instruments, it did determine that each state has the right to require clear and convincing evidence. Missouri's standards in this regard are more rigid than some other sates. Hence the court denied the petition by Cruzan's parents (*Cruzan v. Director, Missouri Department of Health*, 1990).

Another way of controlling one's dying, in addition to the living will and similar advance directives, is provided by do-not-resuscitate (DNR) orders. Patients have a right to require DNR orders in the hospital. These orders mean that no resuscitation efforts will be made during the dying process should the patient's heart and breathing stop. In fact, cardiopulmonary resuscitation was never intended for terminally ill patients suffering from long-term illnesses. Rather, it was meant for emergency interventions when someone suddenly had a heart attack or respiratory arrest. Given the right to refuse treatment, patients and their families may also refuse other interventions such as antibiotics, nasogastric feeding tubes, and intravenous fluids and nutrition (Lynn, 1987; Shannon and Walter, 1988). Interventions such as fluids and nutrition could be said to be death-denying rather than life-prolonging technologies. In the case of dying patients, all treatments should be seen as optional, especially if they might prolong the dying process (American Academy of Neurology, 1989; Cohen et al., 1988; Micetich et al., 1983).

For those patients who have left little or no instructions about what they would like to have done during their dying process, physicians and families may employ the distinction between ordinary and extraordinary means. Ordinary means, in Pope Pius XII's early formulation of this distinction, were those that represented little or no burden to the patient. Extraordinary means were those that were a burden to the patient or the family. Economic considerations were possible in this schema (Pius XII, 1957).

The distinction fell on hard times later, when people began to make of it a normative category: *ordinary means* was to signify those usual medical treatments that were required; *extraordinary means* was to signify those unusual treatments that would be optional (most often, *usual* was identified with items such as food and water, and *unusual* with technologies such as respirators or cardiopulmonary resuscitation). Because of this confusion between normative meanings for the ordinary/ extraordinary distinction, and the original meaning of burdensomeness, today most ethicists and the courts prefer to use the principle of pro-portionality. According to this principle, only those interventions should be used which can demonstrate a proportionately greater benefit than burden to the patient. If the patient is dehydrated but cannot drink water, then intravenous fluids make sense, since the benefit outweighs the burden. If the patient is dying without feeling thirst, and fluids and nutrition merely prolong that dying process, then the interventions are judged disproportionate to the outcome, and are optional. In this in-stance, food and water that are delivered through a medical technology are called fluids and nutrition, to make the distinction between the normal way of receiving nourishment through the mouth and a medical intervention.

The principle of double effect (one action can have two or more effects, one good and the other[s] bad) can be used to justify controlling pain, even if the patient's respiration would be depressed by this control and he or she would die. According to the principle of double effect, one action (using very high doses of morphine to control pain) can produce two effects (control of pain and suffering, and depressed res-piration or death). Even though the second effect is foreseen and an-ticipated, it is not intended. Thus, it is not necessary to keep a dying person in a state of anguish from pain out of fear that high doses of pain control medication might be fatal. The first duty of a physician is to control pain, and the second duty is not to impose his or her values with respect to suffering on the patient (Pellegrino, 1982).

Finally, referral to hospice care (if the disease permits) makes eminent sense when a patient is dying. In hospice care, cruelty is avoided, as are all forms of medical technology which might unduly prolong dying (Lamers, 1986). Even though the case is hopeless, the community can provide the support and personal attention a dying person commands as a duty from the rest of us.

Required Advance Directives

As the staggering statistics about an increasingly elderly population become a reality and our children become a problem for our grandchildren, extremely sophisticated norms for withholding and withdrawing expensive forms of care will have to be in place (Rouse, 1988). These will most probably be based on current guidelines that cover terminal illness, but the major ethical and legal issues today are found in the disputes about certain conditions, such as advanced Alzheimer's disease or permanent coma, that may or may not be seen as terminal states (Hastings Center, 1988). The congressional study by the Office of Technology Assessment is helpful in this regard, as it enumerates the areas in which the application of medical technology to elderly persons causes both ethical and economic problems (U.S. Congress, Office of Technology Assessment, 1987).

Ideally, all decisions to withhold or withdraw care, whether clinical decisions or public policy decisions, ought to be based on the value of enhancing individual autonomy. This would mean that a national policy that respects the value of elders' lives would establish means of allocating care on the basis of self-determination, largely through advance directives. When these are not present, a patient's family should be permitted to influence decisions by constructing the patient's value history, or even by insisting on a minimal quality of life.

I would favor a system whereby all individuals, upon retirement, would be required to execute an advance directive concerning certain optional treatments. This advance directive instrument would be required before receiving one's Social Security retirement payments. The ideal of autonomy can be underlined in such a program by permitting a wide range of choices about the optional treatments. However, because society must be protected from increasing health care costs, individuals would not be able to exercise complete freedom over the choices to be made. A good compromise would be to require that persons make decisions about their care in the future, but that society would not mandate that specific decisions be made. Limits could be placed on certain technological interventions for certain categories of diseases, but individuals could choose which of the available technologies should be used in the event he or she succumbs to specific illnesses (Thomasma, 1989a).

Even though any previous directives would be overridden by the patient's most recent verbal or written wish, the exercise of writing the directive would reveal an individual's wishes (even if the directive were never updated) for families and physicians to act on in the future, and would encourage each individual in society to become more conscious of health care costs and their impact on society, on their own families, and on themselves. Perhaps people could be trained to discuss this with the retiring individual, much as an insurance agent projects the needs of new couples in taking out health insurance. Other family members, as far as possible, should be present.

It is important to keep in mind that any social program that "empowers" elderly persons as Marshall Kapp notes, must also avoid forcing them. Decision making under such a program should be as free as possible, within social constraints. Sufficient information is required to make informed choices, as well (Kapp, 1989b). That is why some assistance in mapping out alternatives is required.

These advance directives could also be updated upon admission to any health care institution, and kept in a national computer registry. In this way, even if one were on vacation in a remote region of the country and were brought to a hospital for an emergency, the advance directive would be easily accessible. As a safeguard, all admission procedures in health care institutions or nursing homes should include, at the very least, a question about the "designated decision maker" for the patient, and legislation should be passed to support the right of such a decision maker to make binding decisions should the patient become incompetent.

Individual Decisions and Social Policies

A social policy governing the limits of access to care for elderly persons should be based partially, as far as possible, on elderly individuals' voluntary altruistic decisions to forego expensive technological interventions. This voluntary effort can be further controlled by a societal decision limiting the use of specific technologies when individuals fall into functional categories that suggest that the intervention would be almost totally useless. The main points of such a social policy would be:

• The right of a person to refuse medical treatment that might prolong his or her life, no matter what his or her medical condition might be. This right should be supported even if the patient is not terminally ill.

- The right of the physician to act as the patient's surrogate against the family when care is requested which is inappropriate (Brody, 1983), both from the standpoint of medical indications and from the standpoint of the patient's own value system (Siebe, 1987).
- A system of categories, to be used for patients of all ages, which would define a range of medically indicated treatments for patients at various levels of function (American College of Physicians, 1988). Outside of this range, no discussion would take place of other medical interventions or technology. No one would be able to "buy" care that was not indicated for their level of function. Everyone in a category would be treated equally. The lower the level of functioning, the less would be the range of indicated treatments to be discussed. Economic considerations nationally could shrink this range, but it would shrink it for all persons falling within objectively described functional status measurements. In effect, these categories would create new default modes for certain clinical conditions. For instance, the assumption that respirators or antibiotics should be provided to persons in permanent vegetative states would be replaced by the opposite assumption.
- The flexibility of the dialogue within the doctor-patient relationship. Each treatment decision, although within the medically indicated range of treatments, would still be individually tailored. Ageist proposals for social policies would destroy this individualized tailoring altogether.

References

American Academy of Neurology, Executive Board (1989). Position of the American Academy of Neurology on certain aspects of the care and management of the persistent vegetative state patient. *Neurology, 39,* 125–126.

American College of Physicians (1988). Comprehensive functional assessment for elderly patients. *Annals of Internal Medicine,* February, 1988, as reported in *Senior Medical Review,* 2 (April), 1.

Beck, J. (1989). Patients could gain from these tools of cost containment. *Chicago Tribune,* February 2, sec. 1, p. 23.

Boyle, J. F. (1984). Should we learn to say no? *Journal of the American Medical Association, 252,* 782–784.

Brody, H. (1983). Ethics in family medicine: patient autonomy and the family unit. *Journal of Family Practice, 17,* 975.

Callahan, D. (1983). On feeding the dying. *Hastings Center Report, 13*(5), 22–24.

Callahan, D. (1986). Health care in the aging society: a moral dilemma. In A. Pifer and L. Bronte, eds., *Our aging society: paradox and promise*, pp. 319–340. New York: W.W. Norton & Co.

Callahan, D. (1987a). *Setting limits: medical goals in an aging society.* New York: Simon & Schuster.

Callahan, D. (1987b). Terminating treatment: age as a standard. *Hastings Center Report, 17*(5), 21–25.

Callahan, D. (1989). Callahan: fundamental changes necessary. *Catholic Health World, 5*(4), 4.

Callahan, D. (1990). *What kind of life: the limits of medical progress.* New York: Simon & Schuster.

Canterbury v. Spence (1972). 464 F.2d 772 (D.C. Cir.), *cert. denied*, 409 U.S. 1064, 93 S.Ct. 560, 43 L.Ed.2d 518.

Carwile, C. (1988). Reclaiming rightful power. *Frontlines, 5*(3: December), 1, 3.

Chicago Tribune (1986). Hospital study finds care disparity. March 10, sect. 1, p. 8.

Chicago Tribune (1989). Group urges tax aid for long-term care. January 10, sec. 1, p. 3.

Churchill, L. (1987). *Rationing health care in America: perceptions and principles of justice.* Notre Dame, Ind.: University of Notre Dame Press.

Cohen, M., Cohen, E., and Thomasma, D.C. (1988). Making treatment decisions for permanently unconscious patients. In J. Monagle and D. Thomasma, eds., *Medical ethics: a guide for health professionals*, pp. 186–204. Frederick, Md.: Aspen Publishing Co.

Cohn, V. (1989). Kinder, gentler nation? begin with health care. *Chicago Sun-Times*, February 12, p. 59.

Coleman, B. (1989). Defining life: new issues sidetrack living wills. *NRTA News Bulletin, 30*(2: February), 1, 8.

Cruzan v. Harmon (1988). 760 S.W.2d 408 (Mo. 1988), *cert. granted*, as *Cruzan v. Director, Missouri Department of Health*, 109 S.Ct. 324 (July 3, 1989).

Cruzan v. Director, Missouri Department of Health (1990). 110 S.Ct. 2841.

Daniels, N. (1985). *Just health care.* New York: Cambridge University Press.

Daniels, N. (1988). *Am I my parents' keeper? an essay on justice between the young and the old.* New York: Oxford University Press.

Eisenberg, C. (1986). It is still a privilege to be a doctor. *New England Journal of Medicine, 314*, 1113–1114.

Engelhardt, H.T., Jr. (1987). *The foundations of bioethics.* New York: Oxford University Press.

Engelhardt, H.T., Jr., and Rie, M. (1988). Morality for the medical-industrial complex. *New England Journal of Medicine, 319*, 1086–1089.

Ethical Currents (1986). Another decision in the Bouvia case. No. 7, May, pp. 1–2, 7.

Fletcher, J. (1988). Setting medical limits. *Update: Ethics Society of Loma Linda University, 4*(1), 2–5.

Franklin, C. (1988). A safety net in need of repair. *Chicago Tribune*, September 15, sec. 1, p. 25.

Franklin, C. (1989). Prognosis poor for medical center. *Chicago Tribune*, August 5, sec. 1, p. 11.

Fries, J.F., and Crapo, L.M. (1981). *Vitality and aging: implications of the rectangular curve*. San Francisco: W.H. Freeman & Co.

Hafka, M. (1985). January ethics events feature Governor Lamm, Emily Friedman. *Frontlines, 2*(1), 10.

Hastings Center (1988). *Guidelines on the termination of life-sustaining treatment and the care of the dying*. Bloomington: Indiana University Press.

Hofland, B. (1988). Autonomy in long-term care: background issues and a programmatic response. *Gerontologist, 28*(June: suppl.), 3–9.

Hope, M., and Young, J. (1988). Resuscitating U.S. health care. *Chicago Tribune*, April 28, sec. 1, p. 23.

In re Bartling (1984, 1986). 209 Cal. Reporter 70; 229 Cal. Reporter 360.

In re Conroy (1985). 98 N.J. 321; 486 A.2d 1209 (N.J.).

In re Jobes (1986). N.J. Super. Ct., Chancery Div., Morris County, docket no. C-4971-85E, (April 23).

Jennings, B., Callahan, D., and Caplan, A.L. (1988). Ethical challenges of chronic illness. *Hastings Center Report, 18*(1: suppl.), 1–16.

Jonsen, A. (1988). What does life-support support? In W. Winslade, ed., *Personal choices and public commitments: perspectives on the humanities*, pp. 61–69. Galveston, Tex.: Institute for the Medical Humanities.

Kapp, M. (1989a). Health care tradeoffs based on age: ethically confronting the "R" word. *Pharos, 52*(3), 27.

Kapp, M. (1989b). Medical empowerment of the elderly. *Hastings Center Report, 19*(4), 5–7.

Kilner, J. (1988). Age as a basis for allocating lifesaving medical resources: an ethical analysis. *Journal of Health Politics, Policy, and Law, 13*, 405.

La Puma, J., Cassel, C., and Humphrey, H. (1988). Ethics, economics, and endocarditis. *Archives of Internal Medicine, 148*, 1809–1811.

Lamers, W.M., Jr. (1986). Hospice care in North America. In S.B. Day, ed., *Cancer, stress, and death* (2nd. ed.), pp. 133–148. New York: Plenum Publishing Co.

Lamm, R.D. (1985). *Megatraumas: America at the year 2000*. Boston: Houghton Mifflin Co.

Lamm, R.D. (1987). The ten commandments of an aging society: the generational conflict. *Vital Speeches, 54*(December), 133–139.

Loewy, E. (1989). Beneficence in trust. *Hastings Center Report, 19*(1), 42–43.

Longman, P. (1987). *Born to pay: the new politics of aging in America*. Boston: Houghton Mifflin Co.

Longworth, R.C. (1989). Britain offers health care reform. *Chicago Tribune*, February 1, sec. 1, p. 10.

Lynn, J., ed. (1987). *By no extraordinary means*. Bloomington: Indiana University Press.

MacIntyre, A. (1988). Whose justice? which rationality? Notre Dame, Ind.: University of Notre Dame Press.

Madigan, C.M. (1989). As citizenry ages, social contract may have to change. *Chicago Tribune*, August 27, sec. 4, p. 1.

Mauro, T. (1988). Blackmun sees switch on abortion. *USA Today*, September 14, sec. 1, p. 1.

McCormick, R. (1989). The Cruzan decision. *Midwest Medical Ethics*, 5(1 and 2), 3–6.

McIntyre, R.L. (1988). Comment: perspective on medical ethics. *Info Trends: Medicine, Law and Ethics*, 4(1), 5–6.

Medical Ethics Advisor (1989a). O'Connor case highlights problem of incompetent patient with no living will. 5(1), 13–16.

Medical Ethics Advisor (1989b). Right-to-die movement takes turn toward hard times. 5(1), 1–16.

Medical Ethics Advisor (1989c). Supreme court accepts Cruzan case, to rule on right to die. 5(8), 97–101.

Medical Ethics Advisor (1989d). System needed to guarantee access to health care in USA. 5(7), 85–93.

Micetich, K., Steinecker, P., and Thomasma, D.C. (1983). Are intravenous fluids morally required for dying patients? *Archives of Internal Medicine, 143*, 975–978.

Millenson, M. (1989). Poll: 90% want key health care changes. *Chicago Tribune*, February 15, sec. 1, p. 1.

Moody, H.R. (1988). Is less better? social justice arguments against life prolongation for the aged. *Gerontologist, 28*(October), 23.

Pellegrino, E.D. (1982). The clinical ethics of pain management in the terminally ill. *Hospital Formulary, 17*(11), 1493–1496.

Pellegrino, E.D., and Thomasma, D.C. (1981). *A philosophical basis of medical practice.* New York: Oxford University Press.

Pellegrino, E.D., and Thomasma, D.C. (1988). *For the patient's good: the restoration of beneficence in health care.* New York: Oxford University Press.

Pius XII (1957). The prolongation of life. *Pope Speaks, 4,* 393–398.

President's Commission for the Study of Ethical Problems in Medicine and Biomedical and Behavioral Research (1983). *Securing access to health care: a report on the ethical implications of differences in the availability of health services*, vol. 1. Washington, D.C.: U.S. Government Printing Office.

Reinhardt, U.E. (1986). Letter of June 9, 1986, to Arnold S. Relman. *Health Affairs, 5*(2), 28–31.

Rouse, F. (1988). Legal and ethical guidelines for physicians in geriatric terminal care. *Geriatrics, 43*(8), 69–75.

Scheer, R.L. (1985). Decisions of life and death require our judges' guidance, Letter to the editor. *New York Times*, October 19, p. 26.

Scitovsky, A.A., and Capron, A.M. (1986). Medical care at the end of life: the interaction of economics and ethics. *American Review of Public Health, 7,* 59–75.

Shannon, T., and Walter, J. (1988). The PVS patient and the forgoing/withdrawing of medical nutrition and hydration. *Theological Studies, 49,* 623–647.

Shock, N.W., Greulich, R., Andres, R., Arenberg, D., Costa, P., Jr., Lakatta,

E., and Tobin, J. (1984). *Normal human aging: the Baltimore longitudinal study of aging.* NIH Pub. no. 84-2450. Washington, D.C.: U.S. Government Printing Office.

Siebe, J. (1987). Are health providers still patients' chief advocates? *Physician Executive, 13*(September/October), 23–25.

Smeeding, T.M., ed. (1987). *Should medical care be rationed by age?* Totowa, N.J.: Rowman & Littlefield.

Society for the Right to Die (1989). The right to die backgrounder. *Society for the Right to Die.* New York: Society for the Right to Die.

Thomasma, D. (1983). Ethical considerations in the care of the dying patient and the hospice concept. *Linacre Quarterly, 49*(November), 341–345.

Thomasma, D. (1984). Freedom, dependency, and the care of the very old. *Journal of the American Geriatrics Society, 32,* 906–914.

Thomasma, D. (1988a). Geriatric ethics. *Journal of the American Geriatrics Society, 36,* 959–960.

Thomasma, D. (1988b). The range of euthanasia. *Bulletin of the American Academy of Surgeons, 73*(August), 4–13.

Thomasma, D. (1989a). Advance directives and health care for the elderly. In C. Hackler, R. Moseley, and D. Vawter, eds., *Advance directives in medicine,* pp. 93–109. New York: Praeger.

Thomasma, D. (1989b). Moving the aged into the house of the dead: a critique of ageist social policy. *Journal of the American Geriatrics Society, 37,* 169–172.

Thurow, L.C. (1984). Learning to say "no." *New England Journal of Medicine, 311,* 1569–1572.

U.S. Congress, Office of Technology Assessment (1987). *Life-sustaining technologies and the elderly.* Washington, D.C.: U.S. Government Printing Office.

U.S. Senate, Special Committee on Aging (1989). *Aging America: trends and projections.* Washington, D.C.: U.S. Government Printing Office.

Veatch, R.M. (1988). Justice and the economics of terminal illness. *Hastings Center Report, 18*(4), 34–40.

Weinstein, M. (1988). Pros and cons of national health insurance. *ACP Observer, 8*(5), 18.

8

Meaning, Aging, and Public Policy

THOMAS H. MURRAY, Ph.D.

When a debate has such a grip on the public imagination as does the one now taking place over the rationing of health care for elderly Americans, it is helpful to step back and ask: Why this debate, with issues framed this way, at this time? Some of the answers are obvious. As other chapters in this volume demonstrate, elderly persons are indeed heavy users of health care. They are more likely than persons in other age groups to have chronic diseases, to be dependent on others for at least some of the basic tasks of life, and to die within a short time. If they live, their lives are more likely to be marked by diminishing vitality; and they are much less likely, now or in the future, to be productive for the national economy.

To put the case bluntly, as many are now prone to see it, elderly people use more health care than younger people, with less benefit to themselves and little benefit (indeed, a net cost) to those of us who are not elderly. So, the argument goes, why not take some of those resources and give them to other age groups?

The argument for discouraging the use of life-prolonging health care among the elderly population is buttressed with controversial claims about the meaning and the significance of old age and death. These claims need to be questioned. The meanings given to aging and the prolongation of life also play a crucial role in supporting—or under-mining—public policies intended to conserve resources by ensuring that they are not used to keep the very old alive.

Images of Aging

The case for rationing rests on terribly important, widely unquestioned, but dubious beliefs about the significance individuals attribute to the later years of life, and about the value of elderly people to society. We are inclined to think of the lives of the aged people among us as having less intrinsic value than the lives of younger people. Seen from this point of view, aged people retire from productive participation in the community's economic life and while away their remaining years in leisurely pastimes of no genuine significance. We say of the elderly that they have "made their contribution"; this may entitle them to our support, but it cannot prevent us from feeling that they are basically superfluous, excess ballast to be hoisted overboard as soon as decently possible.

This image of aging as bringing insignificance and a surfeit of meaningless consumption is not the only image available. One popular counterimage is that of vibrant and energetic aging. As historian Thomas Cole (1983) points out, however, such a conception of aging, while more attractive than the former, is merely the flip side of a narrow and unrealistic perspective. Both conceptions assume that energetic productivity is the key to finding value and meaning in life at every stage. Some people of every age fail to meet this criterion; but the existential realities of aging—diminished appetite, energy, and productivity; the loss of one's age-mates; the inescapable nearing of one's own death—assure that if we live long enough we will each fall increasingly short of the mark.

The policy debate would be deepened if we could understand the roots of the images of aging we bring to it. The debate would also be improved if we saw that other conceptions of the meaning of aging and of the value of elderly persons were possible, indeed lively, alternatives.

The meaning we give to the lives of elderly Americans is inescapably tied to our sense of what is right and just in our public policies affecting them. Moreover, the meaning—or lack of it—that aged persons find in their own lives is both an expression of our culture, and the reason that some voices are now advocating coercive policies to deny life-prolonging technologies to the very old. However, we need to begin with a more fundamental question: What does the end of life have to do with the rest of life? There is no better place to start than with Tolstoy's story *The Death of Ivan Ilyich* (1981).

The Life (and the Dying) of Ivan Ilyich

Despite its title, *The Death of Ivan Ilyich* is more about Ivan's dying than his death; and, more important, Ivan's dying and his confrontation with death are profoundly rooted in his life. Until the last couple of hours, his dying is an extension of the way he has lived, with all the pretense, charade, and shallowness that characterized his adult life. Ivan Ilyich, though only 45 at the time of his death, illustrates the importance of meaning in encounters with illness, medicine, and death.

Tolstoy clears the way by describing Ivan Ilyich's funeral in the first chapter. The story is then free to concentrate on the sort of life Ivan Ilyich lived: "most simple and commonplace—and most horrifying" (Tolstoy, 1981, p. 49). Like countless others in late nineteenth-century Russia, or for that matter, in America in the twentieth century—Ivan Ilyich had lived complacently and shallowly, his reputation and success in the bureaucracy swelling as his humanity shriveled. The son of a government functionary, he "had been drawn to people of high standing in society as a moth is to light; he had adopted their manners and their views on life and had established friendly relations with them" (p. 50). After a young adulthood of mild but measured debauchery ("all done with clean hands, in clean shirts, and with French phrases, and, most importantly, among people of the best society—consequently, with the approval of those in high rank" [p. 52]), he married. Within a year, though, married life proved not always pleasant, so Ivan Ilyich developed what he considered a proper attitude toward it: "he demanded only the conveniences it could provide—dinners at home, a well-run household, a partner in bed, and, above all, a veneer of respectability which public opinion required" (p. 58). At his work in the judicial system, as in his domestic life, he learned "to exclude whatever was fresh and vital, which always disrupted the course of official business" (p. 68).

So went Ivan Ilyich's life, until a pain in his side became impossible to ignore. Physicians were called in. They assumed an attitude of grave importance and omniscience—an attitude Ivan Ilyich recognized as the one he had assumed in court. With repeated assurances that all would be well, they turned aside his questions. Except for overhearing an argument about whether the troublesome organ was his kidney or his cecum, he could learn nothing from his doctors.

Despite his own efforts to deny that he was dying, the truth eventually became inescapable. Now Ivan Ilyich's greatest suffering was caused by "the lie, the lie which, for some reasons, everyone accepted: that he was not dying but was simply ill, and that if he stayed calm and underwent treatment he could expect good results" (Tolstoy, 1981, pp. 102–103). This lie, which "was bound to degrade the awesome, solemn act of his dying to the level of their social calls, their draperies, and the sturgeon they ate for dinner, was an excruciating torture for Ivan Ilyich . . . He saw that the awesome, terrifying act of his dying had been degraded by those about him to the level of a chance unpleasantness, a bit of unseemly behavior . . . that it had been degraded by the very 'propriety' to which he had devoted his entire life" (p. 103).

Trying to understand his suffering and misery and impending death, Ivan Ilyich asked Why—and suddenly received an answer from within, from what Tolstoy describes as the "voice of his soul." "What do you want?" the voice asked. "What? Not to suffer. To live." " 'To live? How?' asked the voice of his soul. 'Why, to live as I did before—happily and pleasantly.' 'As you lived before, happily and pleasantly?' asked the voice." As Ivan Ilyich thought back, the only enduring happy memories were from his childhood, but they seemed to be the memories of another person. The pleasantries of his adult life now appeared "trivial and often nasty." He could not yet bring himself to believe "that life was so senseless and disgusting . . . Perhaps I did not live as I should have . . . But how could that be when I did everything one is supposed to?" (Tolstoy, 1981, p. 120).

Ivan Ilyich's few remaining days were filled with physical and moral agony. The moral agony began with the question "What if my entire life, my entire conscious life, simply was *not the real thing*?" (Tolstoy, 1981, p. 126). After a horrible night, Ivan Ilyich "saw clearly that all this was not the real thing but a dreadful, enormous deception that shut out both life and death" (p. 127). Shortly thereafter, he began three days of continuous screaming.

At the end of those three days, a mere hour before his death, Ivan Ilyich's son grasped one of the dying man's flailing hands as it landed on his head, kissed it, and cried. Ivan Ilyich stopped screaming, and gazed in sympathy on his son and wife. The honest human pity his suffering had inspired in those two, the simple, affectionate act by his son, helped Ivan Ilyich to believe that the worth of his life was not irretrievable and that death was a thing he could accept.

Ivan Ilyich's greatest suffering, and the cause for his fearing death so much, lay in the meaninglessness of his life—that life that Tolstoy described as so simple, commonplace, and horrifying.

Ivan Modernized

Ivan Ilyich's sensibilities are very modern, astonishingly familiar to late twentieth-century America. He was a bit of a sensualist, but not so much as to risk his career or his reputation. If we shaved his beard and dressed him in a blue suit, we would be hard put to tell him from any other bureaucrat or organization man; his attitudes and expectations are perfectly aligned with our own. No mindless romantic or victim of spontaneity, Ivan Ilyich epitomizes the rational, satisfaction-maximizing individual so beloved of economic theory.

When the modern Ivan (the "Ilyich" would certainly have been dropped) became ill, he would have mentioned it, perhaps, at his annual executive physical. His physician, ever fearful of the possibility of a malpractice suit, especially when dealing with a patient who was a lawyer, would have hustled him to an imaging center where Ivan would have been x-rayed, NMR scanned, CAT scanned, and PET scanned. This might have revealed a tumor growing on Ivan's liver, pancreas, or kidney. The fortunate man could then have been bombarded with radiation and suffused with toxic chemicals, and could have had bits of the offending organ cut out. Unless he were exceptionally fortunate, Ivan would have died anyway, perhaps a little later than Ivan Ilyich, but perhaps not. Our contemporary Ivan's treatment would be pricier; it would cost many tens of thousands of dollars. Of course his physical agony might have been alleviated somewhat more effectively, what with new drugs and the (slowly) increasing willingness to use them. However, his moral agony—the sense that his life was not "the real thing" (he would probably choose a different way of expressing this idea so as not to confuse it with a soft drink)—would be just as severe.

"Moral agony" is an odd notion for us. For Tolstoy's contemporary readers, steeped as they were in a religious tradition, the concept might not have seemed quite so strange, though those whose lives resembled Ivan Ilyich's may have been offended at Tolstoy's portrayal of their existence as shallow and meaningless.

Meaning, Dying, and Aging

A great story such as *The Death of Ivan Ilyich* lends itself to many interpretations and is exhausted by none of them. I hope aficionados of literature will excuse me if I choose to focus on it as a parable of the relationship between meaningfulness (or the lack of it) in the life one leads, one's dying, and one's attitude toward death.

How can a life that was so "simple and commonplace" be at the same time horrifying? The answer is simply this: it can be so when the rules by which we live our simple and commonplace lives shrink the human spirit, choke off love and concern for others, and narrow our attention to ourselves, leaving us to the pursuit of small pleasures and especially the avoidance of unpleasantness.

There is abundant scholarship on the concept of meaning, even some on the idea of meaning in aging (see Cole and Gadow, 1986, especially the chapters by Moody, May, and Cole). What I mean by *meaning* is simple enough: it is the purpose and intelligibility that people find, or attempt to find, in their lives. The quest for meaning is the consequence of the ineluctable urge to make sense of one's life—to seek justifications and to construct a narrative, a story of one's life, that makes sense, that makes of it a whole.

The search for meaning has an inner and an outer aspect. Our quest for an inner sense of purpose (the sense that there is after all a point to this life) and integration (the sense of wholeness, that all this seeming chaos fits together) is paralleled by the need for shared public understandings (the ways of life a particular culture offers its members). These available social forms can vary according to one's age, sex, or other characteristics. They can encourage self-absorption by limiting meaning to privatistic concerns. They can set an impossible standard by requiring a vigorous productivity that cannot be sustained in the face of the physical deterioration aging brings with it. Alternatively, they can take into account the existential realities of aging at the same time as they acknowledge that meaning may in part be found through connectedness with other people, in the same generation or in other generations. If most of the outer public forms available in one's culture are shallow, narcissistic, or otherwise thin in meaning, then the individual, like Ivan Ilyich, may grasp a convenient form of life, only to find later that it cannot support him when explicit questions about meaning can no longer be escaped. Facing one's own death is the paramount example of a situation that throws the question "What is the meaning of your life?" smack into your face.

Ivan Ilyich, when asked what he wanted, could only answer, "Why, to live as I did before—happily and pleasantly." That is, he wanted more of the same. However, when the voice of his soul mocked him by simply repeating, "As you lived before, happily and pleasantly?" he was forced finally to confront the ever-increasing emptiness of his life since childhood. After three days of agony, Ivan Ilyich discovered that there were still shreds of meaning in his life. Whatever the implied religious content of Ivan Ilyich's deathbed epiphany, the concrete human event that touched it off was the loving touch of his son, and the tearful stripping away of the facade of his wife's propriety to reveal the simple sorrow and pity within.

It is less important to be taken with the particulars of the indictment of Ivan Ilyich's life, or of how he finally found justification, than to realize that meaning is a crucial element in life, and that the quest for meaning becomes particularly critical when meaning is most threatened, that is, when whatever has functioned as meaning is stripped away through disability, or separation, or severance from the world of economic productivity, or finally by proximity to death.

A Fearsome Dying

It is best to confront our fears forthrightly. What so many of us—young and old alike—fear is an horrific scene such as this imagined one: a woman in her late nineties, dreadfully ill, being kept alive in an intensive care unit by a multitude of machines tended by bustling nurses and physicians. The cost of all this sophisticated intervention is extravagant. The patient, meanwhile, is miserable: semiconscious, in pain, confused by the myriad tubes and wires invading her body, frightened by the masked and smocked strangers who orchestrate all this. Perhaps our patient experiences this as an indignity, a loss of control or integrity. Perhaps she does not want any of this fuss and pain, but in her current state is unable to convey her wishes to those in charge. Her family, to the extent that they are allowed any contact with her, helplessly mourn her suffering and loss of dignity. And while this may last for hours, days, weeks, or even months, in the end it will prove futile: she will die.

This is not the death of any particular person, but there are elements in it of uncountable real deaths. If it is a reasonably accurate reflection of the images you hold of a horrible, wasteful death, then it will serve its purpose. It is the kind of death we fear (and one that Ivan Ilyich, unfortunate as he was, was spared). We fear it for many reasons.

We fear such a death because it is filled with suffering, both physical pain and the sort of anguish that comes from purposeless suffering (Cassel, 1982). We fear it because the aggressive attentions of medicine are not desired but rather are inflicted on an unwilling victim. We fear it because of the indignity visited upon the patient's last days. These concerns are all personal. They reflect our desire never to undergo such an ordeal ourselves or to have anyone we love so treated.

Those who worry about the public policy implications of such dyings, though, tend to focus on another aspect—the waste of resources. A strong desire not to squander money, machines, and personnel on such cases is not exclusively the property of policy experts. I can well imagine the dying person herself experiencing disgust and frustration at what she might describe, were she able, as a foolish waste of society's resources. If she were financially liable for her own care, she might well prefer to dispense with much of it, and preserve more for her family.

Some of what must be done to avert such terrible deaths is already well understood. People must be informed about their right to have a say in their own medical treatment. They must be made aware that methods exist by which their wishes can be made known even after they have lost the capacity to do so themselves. These are the so-called advance directives: the durable power of attorney for health care and the living will. These measures do not pose any fundamental challenge to the meanings of aging or of medicine.

In addition, there will need to be a reinvigoration of a neglected goal of medicine: caring when cure is impossible. The education of physicians must give increased attention to the goals of medicine, and must make caring for patients—with the concern for minimizing suffering and preserving dignity that caring entails—equal in status to curing (Cassel, 1986). When curing is no longer possible, caring becomes even more important. (See chap. 3, "On (Only) Caring for the Dying," in Ramsey, 1970). Physicians must also gain the confidence not to rely on technology when it does not materially add to the care they can give a patient.

The most significant and difficult changes, however, may have to come in the way we think and talk about meaning in aging. But as in the renewed attention to and reinvigoration of the goals of medicine, I believe that there are already strong elements of a deeper and more humanly satisfying sense of meaningful old age at large in our culture, elements that emphasize mutual caring, service, and interdependence. They are more visible in our practice than they are in our public discourse. One consequence of this is that these manifestations of commitment to others can remain half-hidden from ourselves, with their significance unarticulated and unappreciated.

Meaning, Medicine, and the Prolongation of Life

So we come to the question of meaning and the aged, especially the meaning attached to the use of life-prolonging health care in old age. This is the subject of the first half of Daniel Callahan's book *Setting Limits* (1987). To put Callahan's thesis concisely, the aged in need of life-prolonging medical care are at the intersection of two cultural crises of meaning: a crisis in the meaning of aging, and a similar crisis about the proper ends of medicine.

These crises are affected by the mutually reinforcing currents of individualism and modernism. The focus on the worth and the dignity of each individual is not at all at issue here. The problem lies instead in another aspect of individualism: its celebration of each autonomous, rational individual's efforts to choose what sort of life he or she will pursue. Thus, individualism entails difficulties in seriously considering the idea of a substantive good for persons beyond the mere freedom to choose, and in conceiving of individual lives as part of the cycle of generations. Modernism, meanwhile, gives to medicine its unflappable faith in progress and its fascination with technology.

Critics of American culture argue that to be old in the contemporary United States is for many people a harrowing experience in marginality.

No longer economically productive, elderly persons are not valued by their still-productive fellow citizens; many older persons whose own sense of worth was tied into their work feel that way about themselves. The elderly sometimes choose to enter and sometimes are shunted into segregated communities of their own age-mates; in either case, the effect is to wall them off from other generations. A truism, though one worth repeating, is that experience and the wisdom it provides are not valued as they once were; thus, what aged people especially have to offer is ascribed little worth and finds few takers.

Modern industrial culture, centered on a consumer economy, has no place for unproductive members except as future producers (children) or as consumers. While a life of voracious consumerism can provide certain pleasures (as it did for Ivan Ilyich), it fails to nourish the human spirit, and it encourages a concentration on one's self-centered concerns that leads to the individual becoming isolated. It is hard to see how the prototype contemporary consumer could give any better answer to the question asked of Ivan Ilyich: What do you want? More of the same. The same what? The pleasures I can afford, while unpleasant things such as illness and suffering are kept at bay.

Callahan's argument can be expanded along the following lines: The predominant form of meaning available to the aged is a shallow consumerism that has no natural stopping point and no deeper goal than its own perpetuation. This has three mutually reinforcing and baleful effects. First, it provides no sense of closure, of the proper ending of a lifespan. Second, it validates a self-centered preoccupation with one's own amusement and comfort. Third, it promotes an attitude, one might even say a greedy attitude, toward health care—encouraging the individual to feel that whatever might extend his or her life ought to be provided no matter the cost, no matter what resources are thereby denied to other persons, other generations. Medicine's own crisis of meaning leaves it in a position to provide little help. In Callahan's description, "Medicine is perhaps the last and purest bastion of Enlightenment dreams, tying together reason, science, and the dream of unlimited human possibilities" (1987, p. 60). If the only meaning to be found in growing old is to grow older still, then medicine is happy to be enlisted in the cause. When the prolongation of life is the measure of success, and death is defined as failure, the mere postponement of death is equated with success. Such success comes at a cost, however. Callahan again: "A goal of the extension of life combined with an insatiable desire for improvement in health—a longer and simultaneously better life for the elderly—is a recipe for monomania and bottomless spending" (p. 81).

A case can be made that in the contemporary United States, as in other industrialized countries, remarkable increases in life expectancy have created a cadre of older persons who are no longer deemed useful by the industrialized economy. Particularly for those whose worth and identity derived in significant measure from their participation in that economy, aging and retirement create a void of purposelessness, a void that must be filled. Medicine, bless its Enlightenment heart, while it cannot provide more meaning, can occasionally provide more time. Callahan's proposed treatment includes revamping meanings and reconsidering goals. He wants us to establish "[a] goal of aging that stresses the needs of the future generations, not only those of the old, and a goal of medicine that stresses the avoidance of premature death and the relief of suffering" (Callahan, 1987, p. 81).

There are some problems with the argument. While there is, I believe, a good deal of truth to the claim that many older people find the available cultural forms of meaning to be thin and ultimately unsatisfying, a great many people seem to find ample, rich meaning in their older years. Nor do older people's lives necessarily betray signs of selfish preoccupation with their own affairs. Their concern for the welfare of others can take many forms, often but not exclusively concern for younger generations. Moreover, old age need not be predominantly a solemn and austere time. Old people can discover new talents and interests, and form new relationships. Indeed, there can be not merely fun but joy in old age (May, 1986). Finally, there are reasons to think that old people may live lives of much deeper meaning and commitment than even they can at times explain.

In the remainder of this chapter, I will try to describe a more complex view of meaning in aging. I will offer some explanations of why the debate about health care rationing has tended to be framed the way it has, and some reasons to think that all is not so dire and hopeless. Lastly I will try to show the relevance of this discussion about meaning to the current public policy debate. The specter of a coercive public policy that would deny life-prolonging health care to those who are very old seems more controversial and important than all this discussion of aging, medicine, and meaning. However, questions of meaning not only underlie that debate but also set real limits on what public policies can achieve.

Finding Meaning in Aging

In *Habits of the Heart: Individualism and Commitment in American Life*, Robert Bellah and colleagues (1985) discovered a gap between the depth of commitment people actually exhibited in their personal and familial relationships and their ability to explain or justify those commitments. We have, they argue, inherited and perpetuated an impoverished moral language.

Although the tradition of liberal individualism inspires commendable respect for the liberty and dignity of individuals, it also carries with it two major problems for a moral community. First, its emphasis on individual liberty makes discussions about what constitutes a good life problematic. If freedom is the primary good, then each individual ought to be allowed to fashion whatever life he or she wishes, and each person remains the final arbiter of the good life for himself or herself. Second, liberal individualism tends to presume that self-interest is the fundamental human motivation, that the only moral obligations we have to others are those we have chosen, and that our relations with others are much like the relations between nations: governed by contract (usually implied rather than explicit) and motivated by mutual self-interest.

The assumption that all analyses must begin with the presumption of self-interest affects my own field, bioethics. The pervasiveness of this view is visible even in the major theoretical works on justice between generations, such as that of Norman Daniels (1988). His theory presumes that we are primarily self-interested and asks how we would budget for health care over a lifetime. The work is sophisticated and careful. However, there are other important motives for caring for people, even for strangers, through our political or eleemosynary systems (Murray, 1987).

The same presumption infects our thinking about the refusal of treatment. In the many discussions I have heard about the refusal of medical treatment, the right to refuse treatment, based on liberty, is invariably mentioned. Much less often discussed are the reasons why people might want to refuse life-prolonging treatment; and even when the possible reasons for refusing are mentioned, the reasons attributed to the hypothetical patient are almost without exception reasons of self-interest—for instance, the desire to avoid pain or indignity. Rarely if ever do we entertain the possibility that, in part at least, someone might refuse treatment because of concern for others.

An unfortunate aspect of our attitude toward dying people, elderly or not, is a tendency not to take them seriously as moral individuals. The flip side of our compassion is too often a kind of moral infantilization. Certainly, there are brute facts about dying itself, and the modern institutional circumstances of dying, that make it difficult for individuals to assert their moral character. However, not everyone is so blinded by pain, clouded by drugs, or intimidated by hospitals that he or she cannot retain some capacity for moral action. Dying people can be courageous or cowardly, generous or mean-spirited, concerned with their family's welfare or with no one but themselves. To put it simply, people often die as they live (Ivan Ilyich, again). We do people a grievous dishonor when we assume that they are incapable of acting out of concern for others.

Consider a person for whom the well-being of his or her family is important. It is easy to imagine such a person refusing life-extending care that was not overwhelmingly beneficial but would place a terrible burden—emotional, physical, or financial—on his or her family. It would be much harder to imagine the opposite. An act so out of character would lead one to suspect that something had distorted the person's moral judgment.

We should have no less moral respect for elderly persons who are not dying; and we should expect no less from them. The elderly are an extremely heterogeneous group. Among them we find men and women of great nobility and unselfishness, as well as some who are self-centered and resentful. I suspect, moreover, that we will find these types in roughly the same proportions as in any other age group past the threshold of moral responsibility.

To the extent that the contemporary world does not offer elderly persons social roles full of meaning, they are at risk of lapsing into anomie, feelings of worthlessness and resentment, and self-preoccupation. We could undoubtedly do more to support the creation of meaningful roles. However, many aged individuals successfully find such roles in extensions of the activities that have always given them a feeling of purpose and integrity: perhaps nurturing younger generations of their own families, perhaps caring for their age-mates who are more dependent than they.

Erik Erikson, in his article "Human Strength and the Cycle of Generations" (1964), writes of the social contexts in which meaningful forms of life must be grounded, and of the inextricable entanglement of generations. He does not, as some commentators seem to suggest, argue that old people alone have a special responsibility to other generations. Instead, he argues, "Any span of the cycle lived without vigorous meaning, at the beginning, in the middle or at the end, endangers the sense of life and the meaning of death in all whose life stages are intertwined" (p. 133). It is true that the old, while they hold (or still retain) power, have the obligation to exercise that power judiciously: "one generation owes to the next that strength by which it can come to face ultimate concerns in its own way—unmarred by debilitating poverty or by the neurotic concerns caused by emotional exploitation" (p. 133). However, it seems wholly consistent with Erikson's views to say that other generations owe older persons opportunities to lead lives of meaning and value in the face of the existential realities of aging.

Natalie Rosel (1986) has documented how the old people in one community have managed to create meaningful roles for themselves. The residents of the neighborhood Rosel describes have literally grown old together, several into their nineties. Over the years, their sociability has matured into a network of interdependencies. Those better able to cope with the demands of daily life offer companionship and assistance to others, mostly in their late eighties and beyond, whose physical abilities make complete independence impossible. Yet each of these widows or married couples lives in her or their own home. While their lives may seem restricted in space or cramped in routine, they are rich in relationships. The more able among them care, respectfully, for the more dependent. The recipients of care give what they can in return: gratitude, conversation, intimacy, a shared sense of connectedness with distant family or friends.

Rosel summarizes what she learned: "Taking mutual assistance for granted is one finding of this study, the second (and not less important) is that the assistance exists among the elderly themselves. The support network in this neighborhood emerged gradually in response to needs shared by aging neighbors" (1986, p. 233). The response to human need among neighbors is natural and unforced. It requires no calculation of self-interest. By responding to needs, and by participating in a community that is marked by its responsiveness and conviviality, the individual members of the neighborhood make a world of meaning for themselves.

Meaning, Morality, and Public Policy

In the end, the public policies we choose depend much more than is usually realized on the meanings and the moral understandings that underlie them. A recent and widely read book illustrates the strength of a meaning-based analysis, as well as the danger of ignoring meanings when fashioning public policies. Daniel Callahan's *Setting Limits* (1987) begins with illuminating discussions of meaning in aging and the goals of medicine, but then offers and defends coercive public policies without paying sufficient attention to those same concerns.

To put it succinctly, a coercive policy of withholding life-prolonging health care from aged Americans (or any other group) can only succeed if people widely accept its fundamental assumption—that those who are very old should not be given such care. If such a premise were ever accepted, however, a coercive public policy would not be necessary. This idea needs some expansion.

If it became law that the very old were to be denied life-prolonging care, but most people believed that the old had as much right to such care as anyone else, we could expect widespread disobedience of the law. In all likelihood, a thriving black market in life-prolonging drugs and machines would arise; physicians would defy the law in large numbers, and we could even see a modern "underground railroad" ferrying old people to places where they could receive the treatment they needed. The black market could of course be suppressed, but at great cost—a cost measured not merely in dollars but also in damage to our conception of our nation as just. Physicians who resisted could be fined, or banned from practicing, or jailed. We could in short have principled civil disobedience on a broad scale. Unless we have deep and widespread agreement that withholding life-prolonging treatment from any particular group is morally acceptable, a public policy designed to enforce such withholding could destroy civil peace.

If, however, we could come to an agreement that withholding life-prolonging care under certain circumstances was just, we would have no need for coercive public policies. A successful public policy does not necessarily require that everyone at all times do what is desired. If we were able to give support and force to the concern for others—including the desire not to impose unreasonable burdens on them—that people near, death, old and young alike, may often feel, we could realize many, perhaps most, of the economic savings envisioned by proponents of coercive policies, and we could do so without incurring the horrendous symbolic and economic costs coercive policies would bring.

If the overuse of expensive health care is caused by a loss of meaning, the solution is unlikely to lie in a coercive state policy that imposes one particular view of (the lack of) meaning in old age. Even if such a policy could be adopted and, less likely, enforced, its complete failure to address the underlying confusion over meaning condemns it to a brief and unstable existence. People will not accept for long a policy that violates their cherished moral commitments to justice and dignity, or threatens the meaning they find in their own lives.

Those of us not yet elderly see elderly people in two distinct ways. "The aged" exist as an abstract entity replete with stereotypes (often contradictory) and wielding political and economic clout. As such, they may be misrepresented and resented. At the same time, however, they are our parents and grandparents, individvuals with whom we have deep connections and who serve for us as models of how—or how not—to grow old. Erikson's image of "cogwheeling" generations is helpful here. He writes: "The cogwheeling stages of childhood and adulthood are . . . truly a system of *generation* and *regeneration*—for into this system flow, and from this system emerge, those social attitudes to which the institutions and traditions of society attempt to give unity and permanence" (Erikson, 1964, p. 152). The generations live in a relationship of profound interdependency that, at the interpersonal level, Erikson calls "mutuality."

Erikson defines *mutuality* as "a relationship in which partners depend on each other for the development of their respective strengths" (1964, p. 231). Within a family, parents, grandparents, and children live in such a web of interdependencies, each counting on and being counted on by the others for their flourishing. Mutuality functions at a societal level as well. The generations are dependent on each other not only for the physical necessities but also for a confirmation that their efforts have brought forth worthy fruit, and for the promise that a life lived according to the meanings available in our culture can be replete with meaning all the way through.

The point I am trying to make here is easily misunderstood if it is transposed into the moral vocabulary of individualism. I am not opposing coercive age-based rationing because it would violate the moral rights of elderly individuals, though it could certainly do that; nor am I opposing it because it would be harmful to the self-interest of individuals in other generations—though I believe it would be. Rather, I oppose it because it would violently disrupt the relationship among the generations. Such a policy would tell aged persons that their lives are empty of meaning and worth. It would also deprive them of the meaning that comes from seeing the loyal care they have inspired in the generations that follow. Because of the mutuality among the generations, the specter of a meaningless old age would be a threat to meaning at all other stages of life as well.

It may be that those elderly people whose lives are rich in meaning will judge the use of expensive and intrusive life-extending technologies for themselves an absurdity. Their own regard for what they have created, and their conviction that resources would be better used for the regeneration of institutions vital to the well-being of younger generations, may lead many to refuse such technologies. Talking with elderly people convinces me that this is true.

We are left with something of a paradox. To that extent that elderly persons are left with an insubstantial, self-centered meaning for their own lives, a meaning that provides no purpose to their existence other than more of the same, they may cling desperately and selfishly to the last moments of life. A public policy that puts the generations in conflict, that deprives aged Americans of a deep and meaningful connection with the other generations, seems most likely to promote just such a narrow view. We need instead a reaffirmation of our mutuality, our identity as a community of intertwined generations.

References

Bellah, R.N., Madsden, R., Sullivan, W.M., Swidler, A., and Tipton, S.M. (1985). *Habits of the heart: individualism and commitment in American life.* Berkeley: University of California Press.

Callahan, D. (1987). *Setting limits: medical goals in an aging society.* New York: Simon & Schuster.

Cassel, E.J. (1982). The nature of suffering and the goals of medicine. *New England Journal of Medicine, 306,* 639–645.

Cassel, C. (1986). The meaning of health care in old age. In T.R. Cole and S. Gadow, eds., *What does it mean to grow old? reflections from the humanities,* pp. 179–198. Durham, N.C.: Duke University Press.

Cole, T.R. (1983). The "enlightened" view of aging: Victorian morality in a new key. *Hastings Center Report, 13*(3), 34–40.

Cole, T.R., and Gadow, S., eds. (1986). *What does it mean to grow old? reflections from the humanities.* Durham, N.C.: Duke University Press.

Daniels, N. (1988). *Am I my parents' keeper? an essay on justice between the young and the old.* New York: Oxford University Press.

Erikson, E. (1964). *Insight and responsibility.* New York: W.W. Norton.

May, W. (1986). The virtues and vices of the elderly. In T.R. Cole and S. Gadow, eds., *What does it mean to grow old? reflections from the humanities,* pp. 41–61. Durham, N.C.: Duke University Press.

Murray, T.H. (1987). Gifts of the body and the needs of strangers. *Hastings Center Report, 17*(2), 30–38.

Ramsey, P. (1970). *The patient as person.* New Haven: Yale University Press.

Rosel, N. (1986). Growing old together: neighborhood communality among the elderly. In T.R. Cole and S. Gadow, eds., *What does it mean to grow old? reflections from the humanities,* pp. 199–233. Durham, N.C.: Duke University Press.

Tolstoy, L. (1981). *The death of Ivan Ilyich.* New York: Bantam Books.

9

Allocation, Yes;
Age-based Rationing, No

HARRY R. MOODY, Ph.D.

Let me begin by supposing that those who advocate the rationing of
health care on the basis of age are correct in their view about what is
wrong with health care in our aging society: we spend money on the
wrong things, and lavish vast sums keeping debilitated elderly persons
alive, while we spend too little on quality-of-life interventions (e.g.,
home care) for their healthier age-mates and still less on care for infants
and children. Let me further suppose that something approximately like
the "natural life course" urged by Norman Daniels *does* make sense as
a standard for guiding our decisions on the allocation of scarce resources
(Daniels, 1988). I will not further argue this starting point but rather
take it for granted in order to explore what policies may, or may not,
follow from it.

This starting point actually ought not to be unduly surprising or
provocative. The fact is that by the end of the 1980s a remarkable
consensus had emerged among a diverse group of thinkers in the field
of biomedical ethics. Figures such as Daniel Callahan, Normal Daniels,
Margaret Battin, Dan Brock, and Robert Veatch, all philosophers who
might agree on little else, had come to agree that social justice could
require that scarce health care resources be rationed—deliberately withheld—solely on the basis of chronological age. The details and arguments that were offered differ, but these and many other ethicists had
come to this startling and disturbing conclusion.

It would be going too far to suggest that a consensus exists among
all writers in bioethics on this point, but the convergence of the views
of so many distinguished figures is enough to give one pause. The denial

of health care on the basis of age is no longer a "wild" idea and is no longer considered obviously unethical. However, let me go on to say that while I happen to agree with this general proposition supporting the age-based allocation of health care, I disagree emphatically with what Daniel Callahan thinks should follow from it. Specifically, I take issue with what Callahan, in *Setting Limits* (1987) and in his subsequent book *What Kind of Life* (1990) puts forth as two corollary propositions to this main idea. He argues that (1) it is time to begin a national public debate that, he hopes, will lead to a public consensus in favor of withholding scarce life-prolonging care on the basis of age; and (2) we ought to implement this policy consensus by cutting off treatment for people beyond a certain chronological age.

It is with *both* these propositions that I disagree. Further, what I want to suggest is that the debate about the rationing of health care in an aging society has been fundamentally flawed and misdirected. Critics of age-based rationing, as well as its defenders, have confused and conflated what are logically two separate propositions: the plausibility of using the "natural life course" as a framework to guide *allocation*, and the specific tactic of age-based *rationing*.

What I want to argue is that publicly endorsed age-based rationing need not follow from this framework at all. Specifically, if we agree with the global principle—a social justice argument for age-based allocation—we need not necessarily agree with either of the propositions that Callahan urges on us. We can accept a social justice rationale for limiting the expenditure of health care resources without endorsing age-based rationing as the means of achieving this limitation. The "natural life course" is, ultimately, a regulative ideal, an ethical standard for allocating resources. A regulative ideal, however, is not the same thing as a pragmatic principle or a basis for political action. One can adopt very different pragmatic principles in thinking about how a regulative standard should influence practice. Moreover, the choice of pragmatic principles is crucial here if the debate about age-based rationing is to have any positive effect on practice in years to come.

In this instance, *practice* means two things: namely, speech and action. More specifically, it means (1) the terms or the way in which the national debate is framed; and (2) the political means of implementing an age-based allocation policy. In this chapter I want to provide an argument based on pragmatic principles, an argument that leads to a practice very different than what the proponents of age-based rationing urge. I want to examine the ethical imperative of cost containment and look carefully at national health care policies that could be consistent with it. Further, I want to consider what forms of "indirect" political practice are morally and prudentially justified. Finally, I want to look at how our language—specifically, the common use of the term *rationing*—reflects and distorts our ability to consider a realistic course of action.

The gap between theory and practice, speech and action, is at the center of why the debate about age-based rationing has failed, and will fail, to encourage consensus on how to set limits in a publicly acceptable way. For example, it is a curious fact that when Daniel Callahan gets around to the point of telling us just *how* age-based limits will be put into practice, he fumbles badly. He waffles, and he backs away from his original, provocative proposal suggesting that, perhaps exceptions will be made, depending on individual circumstances. We sense that he really does want chronological age to be the sole criterion, and for good reasons: simplicity, consistency, and fairness. However, he also recognizes that withholding treatment in individual cases—for example, withholding penicillin from an otherwise healthy 90-year-old with pneumonia—will prove difficult in practice.

The result is that, at a crucial point in his argument, Callahan begins to make the decision to withhold treatment dependent on a variety of standards in addition to chronological age: the patient's expected quality of life, health factors, the expense of the treatment, and so on. In other words, he gives ground to critics who reject his framework and insist that individual factors alone should be responsible for treatment decisions. As a result of this waffling, readers come away unsure exactly what Callahan would urge in practice. Those who give him the benefit of the doubt suggest that "he can't really mean it" about age-based allocation, while those hostile to his approach simply deride his waffling as a sign that the scheme as a whole is misconceived. In short, the practical difficulties associated with age-based rationing are a stumbling block for any rigid scheme to cut off health resources on the basis of age alone.

For writers such as Daniels and Battin, a different problem of practice arises. They, too, step up to the brink of advocating the limitation of health care on the basis of age, but then shrink back in recognition of the practical dilemmas. Their strategy is different from Callahan's. They suggest that an age-based allocation scheme may be justified in theory but cannot or should not be put into practice until we have a society in which the background institutions are fundamentally just. When that will happen is anyone's guess. No one has identified such a society to date. Thus, Daniels, for example, is very uncomfortable about endorsing the covert practice of age-based rationing in Britain. One reads Daniels's book with the impression that it is difficult, if not impossible, to find any society in the world where age-based allocation could be put into practice within the foreseeable future.

Battin (1987), on the other hand, doesn't like compulsory age-based rationing at all, so she has opted for another approach: promoting voluntary age-based rationing by tolerating rational suicide among old people. Obviously, however, there would be abundant problems involved with putting this scheme into practice. Moreover, since many, if not most, debilitated elderly persons would lack the mental competency for voluntary suicide, there is no evidence that Battin's scheme would actually end up reducing costs. Theory and practice again remain far apart.

Age as a Distributional Criterion

This divergence between theory and practice severely limits the usefulness of all these philosophical proposals for policy makers eager for guidance in making cost-containment decisions. Callahan (1987, 1990), at least, urges chronological age as a clear, simple criterion for the (negative) distribution of health care resources. However, it is not as easy as one might think to say what this actually implies in practice.

There are various ways in which chronological age might be used as a criterion for allocation. Thus, we can distinguish between an *overt* use (the Eskimos putting their old people out on ice floes) and a *covert* use (the British policy on kidney dialysis, never publicly proclaimed). We can also distinguish between a *direct* use (refusing heart transplants to patients over age 75) and an *indirect* use (intentionally not putting an intensive care unit in a nursing home). Finally, we can distinguish between a *distributive* use of age as a criterion (deciding about Medicare coverage for organ transplantation) and a *developmental* use (deciding how much research funding to provide for specific diseases, such as sickle cell disease vs. stroke, or AIDS vs. Alzheimer's disease). In the latter case, we are deciding not about how to distribute present goods but about what sort of goods we want to create in the future. Thus, research on stroke or Alzheimer's disease will benefit the elderly population, just as research on sickle cell disease or AIDS tends to benefit younger people.

The importance of these distinctions is evident as soon as we consider the rules of political prudence that might provide guidance concerning which age-based criteria, if any, could be adopted in practice. For example, as a pragmatic matter, it is easier to use age in a covert, indirect, or developmental way than it is to use age in an explicitly negative way (e.g., to deliberately allow people over a certain age to die). A parallel can be seen in debates about active versus passive euthanasia. Regardless of the ultimate justification of this distinction, no one doubts that, pragmatically, it is easier to approve omissions than it is to endorse outright killing. Similarly, it would be easier not to start up a new program (research on the artificial heart) than it is to get rid of an existing entitlement (kidney dialysis under Medicare). The same point is as true for defense appropriations (to develop new weapons systems) as in medical technology: it's always easiest to stop a project before it gets under way. Thus, probably the most effective way to introduce an age-based allocation principle would be to use it to shape new medical technology for the future rather than to cut off resources in the present. However, there may be other indirect ways of enforcing age-based allocation as well.

If one is persuaded that the idea of a natural life course is defensible on grounds of social justice, then it makes a great deal of difference how this principle is introduced. Proposals to set limits on the basis of a natural life course certainly sound alarming, but some of the alarm disappears as soon as we apply the principle to entitlement programs aimed exclusively at elderly Americans. For example, consider our current Medicare budget and then ask yourself, is this how you would spend $80 billion if you were trying to do the best by our aging population? The answer will probably be no, and that would remain true even if we were to vastly expand the Medicare budget The question then arises, what sort of prudential principles could permit public debate on reshaping the Medicare budget? Even if one accepts the broad principle that some kind of allocation according to the natural life-span principle is reasonable, as I for one am prepared to do, then we need to look at the prudential principles cited above: for example, the distinctions of overt/covert, direct/indirect, and distributive/developmental. Crude images of an age-based cutoff actually miss the point. It is precisely intermediate-level principles and rules of prudence that are most needed here.

National Health Care: A Panacea for Health Care Costs?

At this point, some will consider my argument as it has been presented so far and respond that none of this messy discussion about intermediate-level principles would be necessary if only we in the United States funded and delivered health care adequately. They will argue that a national health plan would eliminate the problem of equity, limits, choices, and intermediate principles.

This is an appealing response, but in practice it is hardly more than a slogan, not a program. Even if the general proposition is accepted, even if we wanted to have the entire U.S. population enrolled in something like Medicare, we would still face the problem of how and through what intermediate, incremental steps it might be possible to introduce a "national health plan" in the United States. Which services would be covered and which would not? What priorities would govern such a system? Unless we simply want to use the phrase *national health service* as a kind of incantation that magically disposes of all problems, we will have to think through questions about equity and efficiency. We should not think that there must be one single solution to the problem of the containment of health care costs. No single approach is likely to do the job, but there are steps that, taken together, could certainly slow the trend toward costly, technology-intensive life prolongation, a trend rejected by those who favor rationing.

We should be skeptical of the idea that there is any single panacea that will reduce health care costs or lead to a more just allocation of resources. Proposals for an age-based cutoff of treatment are defective precisely for this reason. Even if age-based rationing were adopted, it might save perhaps $5 billion per year in health care costs: a substantial sum, but not enough by itself to solve the problem we are facing. We need a combination of interventions to achieve a "remission" in the rise of health care costs in our aging society.

The advantage of a national health plan is not that it would eliminate the need to set limits but, on the contrary, that it might make us face up to the need for limits more directly (Evans, 1985). We should be wary of taking the idea of national health care as some sort of magical solution that would introduce undreamed-of efficiencies, create new resources, or miraculously dispose of allocation dilemmas. It will do none of these things. Judging from other countries' experience—in particular, the experience in Canada—national health insurance might help us rationalize expenditure policies and curtail some kinds of waste. It would sharpen choices for us and put trade-offs into a more uniform framework for comparison. However, it would not, it cannot, eliminate choices or priorities or scarcity. Advocates for aged Americans would do well to remember that national health insurance, judging by other countries' experience, is likely to introduce something similar to age-based allocation. Finally, we must seriously consider the fact that a version of national health insurance for the aged alone is already in existence: that is, Medicare. If we imagine simply extending Medicare eligibility across the entire population, that simple thought experiment should be enough to disabuse us of any fantasy that the American version of national health insurance will somehow make all our problems and allocation dilemmas go away.

If we want to think about collective solutions to problems of equity and health care, then Callahan's and Daniels's concept of the natural life course has a powerful attraction. It allows us to think about the entire life course and about how limits might be imposed on health care in an aging society. It asks us, finally, to take cost containment seriously as an ethical imperative, not simply an economic or technical one. If we fail to devise a means of achieving cost containment through equitable means, we run the risk that limits will be imposed on us covertly and inequitably in the end.

The Historical Moment: Discussions on Cost Containment

Recent proposals by writers on biomedical ethics who favor age-based rationing have appeared in a policy climate obsessed with controlling the costs of health care. Such proposals reflect a profound fear of an aging society and a deep pessimism about the feasibility of cost control. Daniel Callahan (1987; 1990), for example, expresses doubt that, under our current system, any form of cost containment will avert disaster ahead, a disaster fueled by the growth of medical technology, the aging of the population, and a culture of modernity that accepts no limits on life prolongation.

However, the proponents of age-based rationing are vague on just *when* this disaster is likely to come upon us. There is a strange lack of historical specificity in the argument. Has the crisis already started? Will it come when the Baby Boomers retire? When health care spending goes from 11 percent to 15 percent of the GNP? When new technology allows us to keep debilitated elderly persons alive indefinitely? We lack any forecasts for the crisis and have no sense of what forces will be unleashed to constrain rising costs.

Perhaps the biggest problem with the proponents of age-based rationing is the lack of political realism, any sense of what is politically possible in U.S. society. The proposed policy recommendation—that it be *publicly* agreed that some forms of health care would be cut off for people above a specific age—is one it is hard to imagine ever being officially adopted in the United States, whatever one's opinion about the merits of the proposal. Legislative bodies are sensitive to public opinion, and well-organized special-interest groups don't routinely go along with such drastic action. Further, one wonders if there are not other schemes for allocation or priority setting that might allow us to promote fairness, or improve the quality of life for elderly Americans, without evoking the dismaying specter of an age-based cutoff. Even if tough choices must be made, is age-based rationing the only option available.

Unfortunately, the proponents of age-based rationing fail to examine any short-run, incremental policy options. Perhaps philosophers don't feel responsible for addressing these nitty-gritty issues. However, ordinary citizens and policy makers alike need guidance on what kinds of trade-offs and compromises are ethically acceptable, whether at the clinical level or at the policy level. Tax policy, options for managed care, changes in third-party reimbursement procedures, and many other pragmatic options might be feasible.

The absence of prudential or pragmatic judgments here is a serious drawback. As a result, the current debate about age-based rationing is not likely to serve us well as we face serious cost-containment problems in the years ahead. The debate has generated more heat than light. By arousing the anger of old-time liberals, advocates for the elderly, and supporters of pro-life views, Daniel Callahan has provoked an unlikely alliance between these factions and has given them all an easy target: too easy, in fact. At the same time, he failed to address the most serious unresolved issues of justice between the generations that now demand attention. What are the legitimate trade-offs between the claims of present and future beneficiaries under Medicare or Social Security? If we feel that we are spending too much on life prolongation for debilitated elderly persons and propose to reduce those costs, how do we ensure that the money saved would go to improving the quality of life? How will we distribute more fairly the burden of paying for these programs? These questions demand prudential judgments about incremental political actions in real historical time: that is, in the United States in the 1990s. Such intermediate-level principles would link our general ideas or regulative ideals with the pragmatic choices available in the world in which we live.

However, none of these intermediate-level principles are seriously discussed or considered in the debate about age-based rationing. On the contrary, the ethicists cannot seem to move from the level of abstract, general principles (the prudential life-course perspective, the need to accept death or finitude as part of life) to intermediate-level principles that would give us guidance for tactical-level policy choices: for example, what view to take of the enactment and repeal of the Catastrophic Coverage Act of 1988, or proposals for public long-term care insurance, or other options under debate. Must we wait, as Daniels (1988) urges, until all the background institutions of society become just, before the concept of the natural life course can have any meaning for policy judgments? What sorts of trade-offs might be ethically permissible in order to move toward a more just health care system, even if it is not a perfect system? It is not a defect in Callahan or Daniels that they fail to guide us through the latest political wars, but it is a defect that they fail to take their philosophical critique to the next step, the generation of intermediate-level principles that could help inform the current debate. To take that step requires that we openly accept the validity of compromise in ethics and politics (Benjamin, 1990; Pennock and Chapman, 1979).

Politics and Indirect Action

I have suggested an intermediate-level principle already: namely, that indirect rather than direct means should be used. In practice, what this means is that policy should favor age-based allocation, not age-based rationing, of health care. What this comes down to is not hard to understand. *Allocation* means setting broad budgetary or policy priorities (for example, deciding whether to reimburse for a certain kind of service or treatment), while *rationing* means "gate-keeping" to decide whether specific individuals will or will not be accepted for treatment. As a matter of practice, allocation is a way of indirectly setting limits in a manner people are likely to find more acceptable than other methods. This distinction, then, is based on an intermediate-level principle of political prudence, or pragmatism.

Since I urge this distinction on grounds of political prudence, however, it is only fair to look at political and historical experience, which must be the test of any principle of prudence. Are there instances where "indirect solutions" have been used at the policy-making level? Indeed there are, although they are a mixed bag, including both successes and failures. By "successes'" we mean the political legitimation of the decision-making process and thus a consensus favoring action—specifically on "dedistributive" decisions involving cost-cutting. In short, I mean cost-containment measures that work, and are accepted by the public as fundamentally fair and reasonable.

The most striking instance of an indirect solution adopted by Congress has been the use of special-purpose commissions charged with handling "hot potatoes" that legislators would rather than not deal with directly. Successful examples here would be the Social Security Reform Commission established in 1983 and the Military Base Closings Commission established in 1988. The 1983 Social Security reforms responded to a short-run financing crisis but also addressed long-range problems in the system. The recommendations were negotiated behind closed doors and resulted in a grand compromise that left everyone a little bit unhappy but no one seriously aggrieved—not a bad prescription for policy-making success. Legislators who wanted to avoid being on record as "voting against Social Security" found a way to "save the system" and spread the pain among beneficiaries, future recipients, payers of payroll taxes, and the general public.

In the case of the closings of military bases, legislators could not have been expected to vote to close military bases in their own districts. Here we had a classic examples of a "prisoner's dilemma" situation, in which the common good and the optimal good of all parties could only be served by enforcing a deal in which some parties accepted losses that they could never endorse directly. The solution was, once again, a special commission that scrutinized all military bases and came up with a list of those that would be closed. Congress had to accept the whole package on an all-or-nothing basis. The full package was accepted.

However, the special-commission ruse doesn't always work, as shown by the fiasco that occurred in 1989, when Congress attempted to approve hefty pay increases for itself on the basis of a commission's recommendations. The public was outraged, and the vote was rescinded. In this case everyone could understand the issues and everyone had an opinion, usually negative.

Perhaps the most spectacular example of the use of indirect means in making cutbacks is the Gramm-Rudman-Hollings law, which mandates cuts in federal spending at targeted amounts. But is the law to be counted as a success or a failure, in terms of legitimation? Perhaps neither. Because of budget-accounting sleight-of-hand (e.g., counting Social Security surpluses as revenue), the law doesn't really achieve its goals. However, it does enforce a measure of discipline and give legislators the appearance of reducing the deficit. Admittedly, with the use of indirect means comes the danger of hypocrisy and still further evasion of hard choices. This is always a danger with indirect schemes that reflect political prudence.

Closer to the issue of the age-based allocations was the case of the Medicare Catastrophic Coverage Act of 1988, which passed by a wide majority in both houses of Congress after extensive negotiations and a lengthy and convoluted legislative history. National elites, including congressional leadership and key special-interest groups such as the American Association of Retired Persons, expected the Catastrophic Coverage Act to be well received by elderly Americans. They were surprised and dismayed when the legislation ignited a firestorm of protest and calls for repeal or revision of its financing scheme, a relatively progressive income surtax levied exclusively on elderly taxpayers.

The experience with the Catastrophic Coverage Act is significant because it demonstrates the strong negative response aroused when burdens are imposed or cuts are made overtly: that is, when people clearly see what benefits are cut or what burdens are imposed. By contrast, no such public outcry greeted the introduction of diagnosis-related groups in Medicare in 1983, partly because hospital reimbursement formulas are opaque to the general public. In parallel fashion, during the course of extensive debate the Catastrophic Coverage Act was not met with a widespread negative response, largely because senior citizens didn't fully understand the technical aspects of the legislation. They only understood once it was clear that it meant higher taxes and money out-of-pocket for very hazy or uncertain benefits.

The moral of these stories is very clear. When public officials can avoid making overt cuts, they are well advised to do so. Indeed, they take every opportunity to do so; the use of special commissions as a ruse during the 1980s was a popular, and at times effective, example. However, not all means of avoiding or blurring the tough decisions will work. What worked for closings of military bases didn't work for congressional pay raises. In the areas of health policy and aging, the Catastrophic Coverage Act ended up as a catastrophe for legislators. It gained the support of elites but failed to gain legitimacy among older voters, in part because its benefits were directed at a narrow group while its costs were extracted from the more affluent elderly alone. Other critics would point to the fact that the Catastrophic Coverage Act marked a break in the tradition of social insurance. In terms of political legitimation, however, this last point was never the heart of the matter. The key point is that, in contrast to the 1983 Social Security reform, the 1988 legislation did not distribute the pain evenly, and the result did not look like a fair compromise.

The same weaknesses are found in proposals for age-based rationing, which have no chance of ever being publicly adopted by a political body in the United States. Indeed, policy proposals for reordering health care priorities actually appear to have some significant support among elite groups such as bioethicists, health care policy analysts, and perhaps national policy makers. However, public opinion data show that the public at large strongly rejects age-based rationing, or even the need, accepted by elites, to make harsh priority choices. Again, the Catastrophic Coverage Act was a dramatic case of the divergence between elite opinion and public opinion, an instance where Congress and other opinion leaders proved spectacularly wrong.

Is It Time for Covert Action on Cost Containment?

The problem of a divergence between popular and elite opinion is not a new one in democracies. The problem appears repeatedly, and at least one approach to its solution has become popular in our own time in the field of intelligence and military action. I am speaking of course about covert action: the carrying out of low-intensity military or espionage activities authorized by high authorities but not acknowledge to the public. In the case of health care, we can imagine a case in which elite authorities—say, the officials of a national health care system—

agree among themselves about certain spending priorities but do not want these decisions to become public.

In fact, however, we don't need to imagine this case at all. It actually exists. It is a curious fact that in virtually all the countries where age-based allocation practices are in effect—Britain and Sweden come first to mind—these practices were not adopted as a result of widespread public debate. On the contrary, the practices are covert if not to all intents and purposes secret. Covert action in the allocation of health care carries with it a whole series of moral problems, not the least of which is the need for lying and hypocrisy: the systematic suppression of facts that are known to those who carry out the policies. Moreover, there is reason to believe that covert action only works in Britain because of a paternalistic social milieu in which there is great deference to doctors, who can, in effect, manipulate elderly patients and often "cool out" those who might make demands or want to be treated. Morality aside, none of this seems plausible for adoption on American soil.

Let me, then answer directly the question "Is it time for covert action in health care cost containment?" The answer is no: not now, not ever. In national security affairs, covert action may be justified when, for temporary reasons, secrecy is required in a military operation. Even there, however, the Iran-Contra episode reminds us that covert action in a democracy is fraught with danger. Even if other mature welfare states impose age-based rationing covertly, this is not a practice one could responsibly advocate or implement in the United States.

We must note that Daniel Callahan, for one, does not favor covert action. Instead, he urges on us a full-scale public debate, which he hopes, will conclude in favor of age-based rationing. Similarly, Daniels, in keeping with the social ethics of John Rawls (1971), urges that any political principles that are adopted be ones that can be publicly defended. If the denial of treatment on the basis of age is to be justified, he argues, it will have to be publicly espoused and endorsed.

The problem of course, is that it is almost impossible to imagine a situation in which, say, the U.S. Congress or a state legislature would debate and adopt a policy of age-based rationing. We need to remember that Congress was only able to act on Social Security reform in 1983 when public opinion had been whipped up with the rhetoric of crisis. Without an atmosphere of crisis, and without a special commission to take the heat for making the proposals, Congress was unable earlier to solve the financing problem. Just a few years ago, Congress, by a 98-percent majority, passed legislation forbidding the practice of making retirement mandatory at a specific age. Can we really imagine a congressional representative trying to defend to his or her elderly constituents a vote to terminate life-sustaining care for people above a specific age limit? A direct and overt action like this would be impossible. As I have suggested, however, indirect policy options and perhaps intermediate-level principles can be considered in order to reflect the ideal of a natural life course. Age-based rationing, however, will not be one of the practices publicly adopted.

What Is Rationing, Anyway?

My argument so far has resolutely rejected proposals for rationing health care on the basis of age. However, a discussion about age-based rationing eventually needs to consider a fundamental semantic problem: namely, what is rationing? How would we know it if we saw it? Why has the term *rationing* become the preferred word to describe our current predicament with regard to achieving a just system for the distribution of health care resources?

We should begin, I believe, with ordinary language. The most important fact about ordinary language is that we almost never use the term *rationing* to describe the distributional decisions that arise in everyday social practice, including the denial of access to health care. *Rationing*, in fact, is a term that belongs to the discourse of crisis, of extraordinary events. Cases in which rationing is publicly defended are those in which an acknowledged public crisis is at hand: for example, the rationing of butter during World War II or the rationing of gasoline during the oil embargoes of the 1970s. Whenever rationing is announced, everyone is in agreement that a condition of drastic scarcity exists. Moreover, the condition is usually understood by all to be temporary. Admittedly, a practice of permanent rationing might be said to have been in effect until recently in various Communist countries of Eastern Europe, where special stores or long waiting lines, instead of prices, have been used to control the distribution of scarce consumer goods. Let us leave that case aside, however, for the moment.

Don't we ever encounter instances of rationing which are not publicly acknowledged as such? We do indeed. There is evidence that the mature Western European welfare states—Britain and Sweden, for example—practice age-based rationing. This evidence strongly suggests that age-based rationing is carried out there covertly. It is never publicly defended or directly acknowledged (Aaron and Schwartz, 1984).

We do not need to go overseas, however, to find instances of what some would call covert rationing. Within the U.S. health care system, there are several practices that resemble, *prima facie*, something we might legitimately call rationing. These include the following: the distribution of organs for transplantation; the practice of triage in admission to hospital emergency rooms; and extensive queuing for the health care services provided through the Veterans Administration (VA). Several properties of these *prima facie* instances of rationing are worth noting:

1. Organ transplantation involves an intrinsic scarcity: the desired object cannot simply be produced in greater quantity by spending more money, so the scarcity is unavoidable. The scarcity could be reduced by more aggressive policies of organ procurement, but it would still exist. When scarcity is absolute or intrinsic, no one disputes the need to distribute the limited resource fairly; therefore, some type of rationing is preferred. Even here, however, under publicly endorsed allocation policies, one feels that no individual would simply be rejected as a candidate for organ transplantation because of personal attributes (other than medical suitability, such as tissue matching). Instead, people should assume a place on a waiting list. In practice, of course, other considerations, such as money or appeals to public sentiment, do influence organ transplantation. So, in effect, what we have in the United States is covert access rules coexisting with an overt rationing policy.

2. Emergency room triage is also not a matter of turning people away from the health care facility because of some attribute (e.g., age or money) but rather of distributing limited staff time in accordance with need. It is a pure case of rationing by need, which again seems to present few issues of fairness. Again, money or health insurance coverage can play a role here, but officials are usually uncomfortable about that fact, and hospitals, by law, cannot turn away anyone needing life-sustaining care. In the case of emergency treatment, the distributional decision is made at the point of entry into the system. It is not a decision about the availability of a specific treatment, as in organ transplantation. Moreover, the rationale for the distributional decision, or place on the queue, is never publicly announced to the patient in the emergency room, although one might discover it if one asked. Here, too, we have a covert rationing policy.

3. The queuing practice in the VA, like emergency room triage, is a matter not of rejecting a specific class of persons according to their attributes but rather of setting up a waiting list. Need, presumably, plays a part in one's position on the waiting list, but so, perhaps, does the principle "first come, first served," as in other cases of queuing, such as nursing home admission. The effect of a waiting list, as in national health care systems such as those of Canada or Britain, may well be to enforce some broader allocation scheme. However, the origin of the allocation scheme is likely to be not a thoroughgoing health policy but simply the acknowledgment of budget limitations. Unlike other entitlement spending, VA appropriations from Congress are limited to a fixed budget. Once the money is gone, there are no more

services for that year. Thus, queuing arrangements can vary from year to year, just as they vary from one VA hospital to another.

An important feature of these *prima facie* instances of rationing is that they involve a discrete class of goods (organs, emergency room services) or a separate entitlement system (the VA). They are not embodied in a unified health care system of the type that exists in mature welfare states where a unified budget for health care exists. This fact is important because both rationing and allocation are sometimes justified in terms of trade-offs among competing goods. Yet intelligible trade-off decisions are possible only within relatively unified systems; an example is organ transplants versus home care within the Medicare system. In the United States, we have a highly fragmented payment system for health care, and even under public provision, the system is fragmented in ways that make explicit trade-offs or allocation decisions difficult.

Still, there are subsystems of the U.S. health care payment system where strict allocation policies have been put into effect or might be proposed. The Veterans Administration is one; another major subsystem, which has been a prime candidate for strict allocation policies and cost containment, is Medicare. Within Medicare alone, some notable examples of cost containment include the following:

- *The Prospective Payment System*, probably the best-known cost-containment policy, which in 1984 introduced diagnosis-related groups (DRGs), imposing limits on hospital reimbursement and, indirectly, on the length of the patient's stay in the hospital.
- *Price controls on physicians' charges under Medicare.* The New England states and several others have some form of "ban on balance billing" under Medicare—that is, they limit the price of service to the amount reimbursed by Medicare. There are proposals to extend this policy to the national level.
- *Reimbursement limits.* Recent federal legislation, following recommendations from the Hsiao Commission, has imposed physician payment reform. This reform amounts to more than simply a cost-limitation policy, since it regulates reimbursements for medical practice in accordance with a so-called relative-value scale for services provided. Along with proposed "expenditure targets," these reimbursement limits have the potential for seriously limiting expenditures under Medicare and also redirecting where health care spending will go. Physicians' groups have charged that these reforms are the first step toward the rationing of health care.

If this discussion were extended beyond Medicare, we also might look at the state level, where there are other examples: for instance, the denial of Medicaid coverage for organ transplants in the state of Oregon, or New York State's proposed limit on Medicaid recipients' visits to physicians. There are still other examples, wise or unwise, where spending limits—allocation decisions—have been imposed, whether by governments (Oregon or New York) or by insurance carriers, who routinely make decisions about what services to cover or not to cover under reimbursement. None of these allocation examples amount to rationing in the sense described above.

This distinction, and this recent historical experience with allocation decisions, is important because it underscores why the debate about "rationing" is so irrelevant. Indeed, in the recent history of Medicare we have the most instructive example of what cost-containment policies are most likely to look like in the American scene. These policies are, and will be, hotly debated. The containment of hospital costs, the imposition of controls on the prices charged by physicians, and reform of the system for payments to physicians are naturally viewed in different ways by the various interest groups—health care providers, consumers, and third-party payers—concerned with the health care system. DRGs, for example, were initially attacked by interest groups representing not only hospitals but elderly citizens. Recently some critics have charged that the DRG system has actually been ineffective in reducing costs. However, evidence suggests that the prospective payment system, when measured in constant dollars on a per-enrollee basis, has kept Medicare expenditures essentially flat from 1985 through 1989.

Are DRGs, then, a means of "rationing" health care, as advocates for the elderly feared they would be? Or would expenditure targets for physicians inevitably lead to "rationing," as the American Medical Association (AMA) has publicly charged? What is clear in these questions is that *rationing* quickly becomes a label employed to discredit allocation or cost-containment policies disliked by specific groups. Whenever serious cost-containment steps are proposed, *rationing* is the term used to whip up public indignation about where the policies may lead us.

Paradoxically, some bioethicists (e.g., Churchill, 1987) who favor what they call rationing (on the basis of age or other criteria) use the opposite approach. They claim that widespread rationing is already being practiced in the United States—by which they mean, it turns out, simply that access to services is controlled by either the marketplace or by higher-level allocation (reimbursement) decisions. Ironically, one group tries to frighten the public with fears that the specter of rationing is at hand, while another group insists that it is already here! However, this confusion about language, and about the very meaning of *rationing*, simply makes public debate exasperating and impossible.

Let me make the semantic point at issue as precise as I can by giving a definition of the word in question. *Rationing* is a clear and direct limitation of access to an existing scarce good or service at the individual level, when the limit is imposed according to some categorical criteria other than the market.

How, then, do we judge the currently prevailing cost-containment policies? Are they justified because they don't (yet?) amount to "rationing?" It is not my purpose to defend DRGs or any other specific form of cost containment. Individual proposals for allocation or cost containment may be wise or unwise, and should be debated in terms of equity and efficiency. My purpose is simply to indicate that recently proposed or initiated allocation policies within the age-tested Medicare system are

1. Potentially effective in restraining costs (whether in desirable ways is another matter);
2. Capable of being successfully (i.e., "legitimately") accepted in the American political economy of health care; and
3. Analytically different in kind from actual rationing.

The last point is crucial. None of these different allocation policies, or still others that I would favor based on the "natural life course" (e.g., the limitation of organ transplantation under Medicare) resembles rationing. To be sure, these policies may permit or entail gate-keeping behavior at lower levels in the health care system: for example, reimbursement according to DRGs may mean that some individuals don't get to stay in hospitals as long as they want to or perhaps as long as they should. Then too, since all of these cost-containment steps were undertaken within the Medicare system, none of them are comparable to the age-based rationing currently debated. People over an arbitrary age are not denied treatment. Instead, allocation decisions taken at the highest level turn out to entail painful choices, even denial of service, at lower levels.

The resulting pattern of denial is indirect and is therefore often unpredictable in its consequences. For just that reason, it may be easier to legitimate or defend to the public. However, public legitimation does not entail that allocation policies should be beyond criticism on the basis of intermediate-level principles. On the contrary, the whole purpose of this critique of age-based rationing is to insist that we need intermediate-level principles to guide public choice and public debate. To describe the present system, with its indirect pattern of denial, is not necessarily to justify it; it is simply to argue that this pattern is far, far different form anything resembling rationing, and further, that this *indirect* manner of enforcing policy decisions is the one we are likely to be facing for the foreseeable future. A waiting list, for example, is a very different practice from the age-based rationing urged by Callahan and others.

The same point can be made about other indirect allocation schemes, such as altering incentives under a relative value scale or changing reimbursement policies; but none of these schemes at all resembles "rationing" as it is customarily understood: namely, as part of the rhetoric of crisis. In recent years we have seen a growing literature that invokes the specter of rationing when, in truth, what is really at issue is whether we can or should adopt strict policies for health care allocation (Blank, 1988). As I have argued, the distinction between rationing and allocation is partly rhetorical but is also partly a matter of strategy and practical political judgment.

From the standpoint of prudence, it makes a great difference how we frame this problem. What we are likely to see in the future is not age-based rationing, but indirect means of enforcing cost-containment policies. Whether we label this pattern as "muddling through," as the "tyranny of small decisions," or as an immoral evasion of fundamental choices, it is wise to deal with the ethical dilemmas presented by it and by allocation decisions in the present system. It is unwise to be distracted by debates about "rationing," whether on the basis of age or other criteria.

When we turn to the real world of health care allocation, we find a picture that is very confused. Where rationing exists, we can speak of a "clear and direct limitation of access," which simply means that we can discern a predictable pattern in the distributional scheme, whether or not that pattern is publicly acknowledged. As a rule, the pattern will be discernible by the policy makers (as in Britain), and it becomes a normal part of their calculations. In other situations, however, the pattern of access or denial may be more opaque or concealed. Hence, we can speak of overt versus covert rationing.

Now opaqueness, even mystification, is one thing; chaos is something else again. Both , unfortunately, are realities of administrative and political life; and a pattern of practice that distributes resources in unpredictable or chaotic ways cannot plausibly be described as rationing. The pattern may be a way of coping with a temporary shortage. It may represent social prejudice or bureaucratic expediency: for example, the practice of locating a social service office in an inaccessible place, or curtailing its office hours. The effect, intended or not, may well be to reduce the rate of service. Such practices can, and should, be subjected to ethical scrutiny, but it does not seem plausible to describe them as rationing, nor does such labeling help to clarify the debate about what should be done in the face of those practices or the scarcities that engender them.

This point is important because we need to recognize a large degree of "overdetermination" in social decisions of all kinds. In the health care system in particular, as practitioners, administrators, and policy makers try to cope with scarcity, they are likely to act with a high degree of improvisation and a low degree of coordinated policy. In a federal system, in a mixed economy, this state of affairs is only to be expected. Chaos, rather than conspiracy, is likely to be the order of the day. That is a fair description of the fragmented American health care system as it has evolved to the present.

For just that reason, when steps are taken to limit access to health care, we should resist the temptation to extend the term *rationing* in some sort of vague or elastic fashion to cover this kind of improvisation. In fragmented systems, responsibilities are diffused: everybody is in charge, and nobody is in charge. This diffusing of the locus of responsibility for social choice is precisely what the private marketplace achieves, and it is one of the reasons marketplace decisions are often resistant to ethical challenge. For example, it is simply implausible to say that food corporations ration the availability of supermarkets in ghettoes. Nor should we describe the "redlining" practices of banks in terms of rationing. We might well disapprove of these practices and subject them to ethical challenge, but they are not plausibly described as rationing, even if carried out by a public authority.

What, then, about the indirect effects of tight budgetary limits on expenditures in a specific public program? This is hardly an unusual state of affairs: most public programs routinely operate under budget limits. However, we would hardly think of a cut in the annual subsidy for Amtrak as a form of rationing of railroad service in the United States. It may be that because of budget cuts, Amtrak will in fact decide to discontinue service to a specific city, imposing hardship (justified or not) on that locality, but Amtrak will not thereby ration its services. We might not like the decision; we might debate it; but the allocation decision here isn't a case of rationing.

On the other hand, suppose Amtrak decided to reduce its service to City X to one train per week, and then introduced a lottery or used the alphabetical order of names or some such scheme to decide who would get to ride the train. Then we would indeed start to describe the scheme as a rationing of railroad service. Why? Because now we are controlling access to the scarce service at the individual level. By contrast, when the decision is made at a collective level, it is more properly described as allocation, not rationing.

Finally, when authorities at a higher level have made an allocation decision, it is always possible that lower-level officials may be tempted to introduce rationing, or other gate-keeping measures, as a means of coping with the shortage signalled by the higher-level budgetary or policy decisions. They may do it covertly (as in emergency room triage) or overtly (as with organ transplantation). However, rationing, in the strict sense of the term, represents only one means of making allocation decisions.

There are further analogies in health care. Medicare, for instance, does not pay for any form of dental care, yet no one has described the denial as a form of rationing. Similarly, we might decide as a matter of allocation policy that Medicare would not now, or perhaps not ever, pay for the availability of the artificial heart. Some people would die as a result of that decision. It might or might not be the right policy decision; but it would not be a form of rationing because we are not controlling individual access but are instead making collective decisions, at a higher, aggregate level: in short, allocation decisions.

What about intermediate cases, we may ask? Let us return to the Amtrak example. Suppose subsidies are cut and train service is curtailed. Now, access to the train is available on a first-come, first-served basis. Does the use of a waiting list count as rationing? Not necessarily. Do we ordinarily describe the practice of making moviegoers wait on lines for popular movies as a method of rationing seats? No, but if the practice became a customary state of affairs, we might be inclined to. Then we would be in a situation where individual access would be controlled, day by day, according to nonmarket criteria (place on the line). Once again, we can look to examples of the same problem in the area of health care. Consider the case of the admission of patients to desirable nursing homes. This is a case where neither pure market forces nor pure categorical criteria (e.g., need, or the waiting list) dominate the decision. Actual admissions decisions are usually blurred and diffuse, even if the shortages are real. The case falls into a gray area.

One further point about the definition of rationing offered here. The purpose of a definition is not to depict the fundamental nature of rationing for all time but simply to suggest that we have here a broad "family resemblance" among different uses of a concept. Certain ideas (limit, scarcity) are embedded in social practices (breakdown of markets, waiting lists). Above all, it is essential to remember that rationing is, all too often, purely a rhetorical or pejorative term that quickly loses its usefulness unless we attend carefully to the actual social practice in question and the logic of the decisions that must be made.

The prevailing social background to any use of the rhetoric of rationing, of course, is the existence of scarcity or shortages. One solution to shortages, urged by defenders of the marketplace, is obvious:

charge a price that clears the market, thus avoiding the need for rationing. Indeed, a most important feature of rationing is that it is a method of distributing resources outside the market system. In our market economy, rationing is a signal that something is drastically wrong, that the distribution system has broken down and a crisis is at hand. However, the odd fact is that we almost never encounter instances of rationing around us. The point of bringing the term into the debate lies in its rhetorical force. I believe that the term *rationing* is almost always a red herring that serves to confuse the debate on whether a specific allocation policy is wise or desirable.

In the case of Daniel Callahan's proposal for overt, publicly endorsed rationing on the basis of age, we do have a proposal that is much more than rhetoric. It is clear that here we really do have a proposal for rationing in the full and literal sense of the term. However, even if the practice of age-based rationing—say, along the lines urged by Norman Daniels—were ethically justified, the real question is not whether a hypothetical rationing scheme is ethically right but whether it is prudent or feasible. The answer, I believe, is no. Such proposals, as they stand, are unnecessary, impracticable, and unwise.

An age-based allocation scheme, however, is eminently prudent and feasible. The proof of this is the fact that 25 years ago in the United States we introduced an age-based allocation scheme (Medicare), and the program has won wide public acceptance. Any age-based allocation scheme approves some services and denies approval for others. To say yes to some things is to say no to others. There is nothing to prevent us from making the pattern of approval and denial consistent with a framework of the prudential or "natural" life course or with some other regulative ideal. However, we will need intermediate-level principles of prudence to make the complete argument on behalf of any revised approach to allocation.

Despite pessimistic claims that no efforts to achieve cost containment have been successful, I believe there is evidence that cost containment can achieve success. In the United States we have introduced some partially successful cost-containment measures (DRGs) and are likely to devise others. The best proof that age-based allocation schemes are prudent and feasible is the experience of other countries. Virtually all mature welfare states make decisions about allocation priorities and enforce these decisions through production decisions, access controls, definition of services, and compensation for health care providers. In some cases these countries limit access to selected services for people past a certain age. They always set limits, as they must; but they do so without the crisis rhetoric of rationing.

Most of these allocation schemes result in indirect limits on what services will actually be available to those who want them. Inevitably, many of those judgments have consequences for people of different ages. For example, long waiting lists are more of a hardship for people of advanced age and limited life expectancy. A preference for providing more "soft" services (e.g., home care) than "hard" services (e.g., technology-intensive medicine) means that some acutely ill people, mostly elderly, will die who would otherwise live. The wealthy among them may even travel to the United States to arrange organ transplants or may "buy out of" the public system in their own country. Such "buy-outs," within limits, do not necessarily compromise the basic fairness of those public systems of provision.

Last but not least, those systems of public provision in mature welfare states also include, in some cases at least, schemes for covert age-based rationing, of which the most famous is the rationing of kidney dialysis in Britain. However, there is no reason to believe that age-based rationing, covertly practiced, is an unavoidable element of a system that accepts age-based allocation. It is possible to have age-based allocation, along the lines of the "natural life course" or other principles urged by bioethicists, without approving either an overt or covert form of age-based rationing. The key to whether we achieve it lies not in the realm of theory but in political prudence, an altogether different domain (Garver, 1987).

Indeed, I would argue finally that the debate about age-based rationing distracts our attention from what is in reality the more serious debate: namely, how to prudently introduce cost controls and how to distribute the burden of paying for health care in an aging society. All of the serious policy debates of the 1980s, from DRGs (introduced in 1984) to the Medicare Catastrophic Coverage Act of 1988, revolved around cost containment and tax policy. These debates involve major issues of intergenerational equity that are now inescapable (Kingson et al., 1986; Longman, 1987; Moody, 1988). These are serious debates, and they require analysis of the problem of justice between generations. The debate about age-based rationing is not, in this sense, a "serious" debate at all, because it is not a debate about a proposal that anyone could seriously anticipate becoming law.

Philosophers, Theory, and Practice

Why, then, has the debate about age-based rationing so captured public attention? It has captured our attention because it seems to promise a quick fix for a problem—cutting expenditures for health care—that has proved extraordinarily difficult for our political system. In this respect, Callahan's proposal for categorical age-based rationing resembles Reagan's "Star Wars" program, the flat tax, and world federalism: it is a startling proposal that has few prospects for actually working in practice.

However, wild ideas are not altogether to be dismissed. In the perspective of history, "Star Wars" may prove to have been a significant episode on the road to arms control. In the same way, crankish proposals for the flat tax were turned aside, but tax reform eventually became law in the Tax Reform Act of 1986. World federalism, too, retains its adherents; but for most of us, diplomacy and negotiation represent a more promising, and more prudent, path to world order.

What I mean to suggest by these examples is that philosophers, such as Callahan, Daniels, and others, who propose speculative ideas and theoretical models, can do us a service by stimulating public debate. Once the debate gets under way, however, it appears that the philosophers have little to contribute to the detailed resolution of problems. The very model of philosophical discourse today, even when it seems superficially practical, increasingly departs from the discourse of politics and practice (Mapel, 1989). Philosophical discourse has long needed an adequate account of the importance of compromise in the real world of political action (Benjamin, 1990; Pennock and Chapman, 1979). As a result, philosophical discourse is often lacking in prudence or practical wisdom.

This state of affairs is not new. Plato, in his younger days, wrote *The Republic* (1887b), which was a portrait of the ideal city-state. In his old age, however, he recognized that his ideal was too far from ordinary experience, and he went on to write *The Laws* (1887a), a detailed prescription for statecraft in a "second-best" world where humanity is accepted for what it is: namely, imperfect. Today, however, few people read *The Laws*, while everyone knows *The Republic*. Moreover, when Plato himself tried his hand at practical statecraft, on the island of Syracuse, he botched the job and barely escaped with his life.

Philosophers, I would insist, have much to contribute in helping us to think about ideals and purposes. The concept of a "natural life course," I believe, provides a framework in which a practical debate might unfold. The ideal of the natural life course reminds us, in the biblical phrase, to "number our days." It counsels us that finitude is inextricably bound up with our human state and insists that no ideal of justice can prevail unless it recognizes the cycle of generations and the limits of life and death. When the practical debate is anchored in this existential understanding, we may finally have a public dialogue worthy of the serious questions that face us in the future. In the meantime, we need all the practical wisdom we can get to guide us in the "second-best" world where political prudence is needed now more than ever.

References

Battin, M.P. (1987). Choosing the time to die: the ethics and economics of suicide in old age. In S. Spicker, ed., *Ethical dimensions of geriatric care*, pp. 161–189. Dordrecht, Holland: D. Reidel.

Benjamin, M. (1990). *Splitting the difference: compromise and integrity in ethics and politics*. Lawrence: University of Kansas Press.

Blank, R.H. (1988). *Rationing medicine*. New York: Columbia University Press.

Callahan, D. (1987). *Setting limits: medical goals in an aging society*. New York: Simon & Schuster.

Callahan, D. (1990). *What kind of life: the limits of medical progress*. New York: Simon & Schuster.

Churchill, L.R. (1987). *Rationing health care in America: perceptions and principles of justice*. Notre Dame, Ind.: University of Notre Dame Press.

Daniels, N. (1988). *Am I my parents' keeper? an essay on justice between the young and the old*. New York: Oxford University Press.

Evans, R. (1985). Illusions of necessity: evading responsibility for choices in health care. *Journal of Health, Politics, Policy and Law 10*, 439–467.

Garver, E. (1987). *Machiavelli and the history of prudence*. Madison: University of Wisconsin Press.

Kingson, E.R., Hirshorn, B.A., and Cornman, J.M. (1986). *Ties that bind*. Washington, D.C.: Seven Locks Press.

Longman, P. (1987). *Born to pay*. Boston: Houghton, Mifflin Co.

Mapel, D. (1989). *Social justice reconsidered*. Champaign-Urbana: University of Illinois Press.

Moody, H.R. (1988). Generational equity and social insurance. *Journal of Medicine and Philosophy, 13*(1), 31–56.

Pennock, J.R., and Chapman, J. (1979). *Compromise in ethics, law, and politics*. New York: New York University Press.

Plato (1987a). *The laws*. In M.A. Jowett, ed., *The dialogues of Plato*, vol. 4, pp. 1–480. New York: Charles Scribner's Sons.

Plato (1987b). *The republic*. In M.A. Jowett, ed., *The dialogues of Plato*, vol. 2, pp. 1–452. New York: Charles Scribner's Sons.

Rawls, J. (1971). *A theory of justice*. Cambridge, Mass.: Harvard University Press.

Index

Designed by Ann Walston

Composed by Easton Publishing Services, Inc.
in Sabon text with Meridien display

Printed by The Maple Press Company
on 60-lb. Glatfelter Eggshell Offset